Radionuclides in Nephro-Urology

Contributions to Nephrology

Vol. 79

KARGER

Basel · München · Paris · London · New York · New Delhi · Bangkok · Singapore · Tokyo · Sydney

7th International Symposium on Radionuclides in Nephro-Urology, Williamsburg, Va., May 7–10, 1989

Radionuclides in Nephro-Urology

Volume Editors
M. Donald Blaufox, Bronx, N.Y.;
Norman K. Hollenberg, Boston, Mass.;
Claude Raynaud, Orsay, France

70 figures and 31 tables, 1990

KARGER

Basel · München · Paris · London · New York · New Delhi · Bangkok · Singapore · Tokyo · Sydney

Contributions to Nephrology

Library of Congress Cataloging-in-Publication Data
International Symposium on Radionuclides in Nephro-urology (7th: 1989: Williamsburg, Va.)
Radionuclides in nephro-urology/7th International Symposium on Radionuclides in Nephro-urology, Williamsburg, Va., May 7–10, 1989; volume editors, M. Donald Blaufox, Norman K. Hollenberg, Claude Raynaud.
(Contributions to nephrology; vol. 79)
Includes bibliographical references.
1. Kidneys – Radionuclide imaging – Congresses. 2. Urinary organs – Radionuclide imaging – Congresses. I. Blaufox, M. Donald. II. Hollenberg, Norman K. III. Raynaud, C. (Claude) IV. Title. V. Series: Contributions to nephrology; v. 79.
[DNLM: 1. Kidney – radionuclide imaging – congresses. 2. Urinary Tract – radionuclide imaging – congresses. W1 CO778UN v. 79/WJ 302 I615r 1989]
RC904.5.R32I57 1989 616.6′107575 – dc20 DLC
ISBN–3–8055–5073–1

Bibliographic Indices
This publication is listed in bibliographic services, including Current Contents® and Index Medicus.

Drug Dosage
The authors and the publisher have exerted every effort to ensure that drug selection and dosage set forth in this text are in accord with current recommendations and practice at the time of publication. However, in view of ongoing research, changes in government regulations, and the constant flow of information relating to drug therapy and drug reactions, the reader is urged to check the package insert for each drug for any change in indications and dosage and for added warnings and precautions. This is particularly important when the recommended agent is a new and/or infrequently employed drug.

Printed in Switzerland by Thür AG Offsetdruck, Pratteln
ISBN 3–8055–5073–1

Contents

Renal Function

Renal Imaging

Pediatrics

Hypertension

Special Reports of Collaborative Studies in Captopril Renography

Acknowledgements

The organizers wish to thank the following institutions for their generous support of this conference and proceedings:

Major Sponsors

Hypertension Research Laboratory Foundation, New York, New York, USA
Mallinckrodt, Inc., St. Louis, Missouri, USA
Nihon Medi-Physics Co. Ltd., Tokyo, Japan
Squibb Diagnostic, Princeton, New Jersey, USA

Sponsors

Elscint Inc., Boston, Massachusetts, USA
W.B. Saunders Co., Philadelphia, Pennsylvania, USA
G.D. Searle and Co., Skokie, Illinois, USA

Contributors

Boehringer Ingelheim Pharmaceuticals, Inc., Ridgefield, Connecticut, USA; Mallinckrodt Diagnostic, Vienna, Austria; Merrell Dow Research Institute, Cincinnati, Ohio, USA; Frosst Pharmaceuticals, Division of Merck Frosst Canada, Inc., Quebec, Canada; Pfizer Pharmaceuticals Co., New York, New York, USA; Sandoz Pharmaceuticals Co., East Hanover, New Jersey, USA; Boehring Institut Ges. m.b.H., Vienna, Austria; Capintec Inc., Ramsey, New Jersey, USA; Danish Society of Uroradiology, Copenhagen, Denmark

Preface

During the week of May 7, 1989, one hundred twenty physicians and scientists from nineteen countries around the world gathered to discuss the role of nuclear medicine procedures in the diagnosis and evaluation of diseases of the genitourinary system. A further emphasis was placed on the unique role of radiolabeled tracers in the interpretation of the physiology and functioning of the kidney. This was the seventh such symposium in a series of meetings which began in 1968 in Liège, Belgium. The meetings have been held throughout the world in Liège; New York, N.Y., USA; West Berlin, Germany; Boston, Mass., USA; London, England; Lausanne, Switzerland, and most recently in Williamsburg, Va., USA. Each of these meetings is noteworthy for the great interest and wide backgrounds of the participants. Attendees at the most recent meeting included physiologists, chemists, urologists, nephrologists, pediatricians, and nuclear medicine physicians, as well as representatives from a number of other specialties.

The medical community has experienced renewed interest in the potential role of nuclear medicine procedures in kidney disease, with the introduction of captopril to the differential diagnosis of renovascular hypertension. The popularity of this area of endeavor has varied greatly in the United States from periods of great interest to periods of little interest. However, the use of captopril has excited the imagination of the nephrologists and the introduction of a technetium-labeled tubular agent, technetium-MAG_3, has stimulated the nuclear medicine community once again. This interest has been much more steady and less vicarious in Europe where there has been an ongoing and active application of radionuclides in nephrology throughout the years. Technetium-MAG_3, which we are hoping to have available next year in the United States, has been used routinely for several years now in the major European centers.

More than 100 abstracts were received to fill only 35 places on the program. The very high quality of the material necessitated the addition of another 36 poster sessions to make possible the fullest communication.

It is hoped that the publication of these proceedings will serve a useful purpose for those persons who attended the meeting and wish to have a permanent reference. The material may also serve as a reference source for ongoing work for those persons who for various reasons could not attend the meeting.

The organizers of the meeting wish to thank all of the participants for their healthy enthusiasm, which helped to make the meeting a success, and thank those firms and organizations which contributed funds to the meeting to insure its financial solvency.

The Eighth Meeting on Radionuclides in Nephro-Urology will be held somewhere in the United Kingdom under the chairmanship of Dr. Patrick O'Reilly, with Drs. Andrew Taylor and Leonard Rosenthall serving as co-chairpersons. It will be held approximately three years from the date of the Williamsburg meeting at a place and time to be announced.

We look forward to seeing all of the participants in the Seventh international meeting at the Eighth and we hope to see many new faces and hear of many new developments.

Scientific Committee

A. Bischof-Delaloye, MD, Switzerland
A. Basu, MD, India
Joseph Nally, Jr., MD, USA
Patrick O'Reilly, MD, England
Georg Riccabona, MD, Austria
Leonard Rosenthall, MD, Canada
Andrew Taylor, Jr., MD, USA
Henrik Thomsen, MD, Denmark

Chairmen

M. Donald Blaufox, MD, PhD, USA
Norman K. Hollenberg, MD, PhD, USA
Claude Raynaud, MD, France

Special Invited Paper

Blaufox MD, Hollenberg NK, Raynaud C (eds): Radionuclides in Nephro-Urology.
Contrib Nephrol. Basel, Karger, 1990, vol 79, pp 1–10

Angiotensin, ACE Inhibition, and the Renal Circulation: Pathogenesis of Nonmodulation in Essential Hypertension

Norman K. Hollenberg, Gordon H. Williams

Departments of Medicine and Radiology, Harvard Medical School and Brigham and Women's Hospital, Boston, Mass., USA

Despite long-standing interest in the role of the kidney in the pathogenesis of essential hypertension, until recently that role has remained obscure. The thrust of this essay will be to organize a growing body of evidence which indicates that an abnormality of the kidney, and the adrenal, involving disordered regulation through the renin-angiotensin system, is responsible for the pathogenesis in about 45% of patients – a discrete subgroup that may be the most common cause of hypertension. That fundamental abnormality leads to disordered renal sodium handling and sodium-sensitive hypertension, abnormalities in the renal vascular response to changes in sodium intake and to angiotensin II, blunted decrements of renin release in response to saline or angiotensin II, and an accentuated renal vasodilator response to angiotensin-converting enzyme (ACE) inhibition. Because ACE inhibition increases renal blood flow substantially more in these patients than it does in normal subjects or other essential hypertensives, nuclear medicine techniques might prove useful in identifying such patients as a by-product of the captopril renogram, in search of renovascular hypertension. ACE inhibition also restores to normal the renal vascular and adrenal response to angiotensin II, renin release in response to angiotensin II, renal sodium handling – and ultimately blood pressure. Finally, and perhaps most intriguing, similar abnormalities have been found in 50% of the normotensive offspring of patients with essential hypertension and evidence is accruing to indicate that the abnormality is inherited as a Mendelian dominant.

Sodium and Renal Vascular Responses to Angiotensin II

Dahl [1] in a 1963 review of metabolism in hypertension was puzzled by five then recent publications, which described a paradoxical, natriuretic response to angiotensin II associated with a blunted or absent renal vascular response in some patients with essential hypertension. He noted the parallel with hepatic cirrhosis. Since then, the mechanism in cirrhosis has become clear [2]. The paradoxical natriuresis reflects the effects on renal sodium handling of the pressor response, when the renal vascular bed can no longer respond to angiotensin II because of angiotensin-mediated renal vasoconstriction.

During that time, two separate lines of investigation on disordered control of the renal blood supply [3] and the adrenal [4] with shifts in state of sodium balance led to the recognition that both abnormalities occur in the same patient [5]. This followed recognition of a highly predictable shift in renal vascular and adrenal responses to angiotensin II with changes in sodium intake: the renal vasculature is more sensitive to angiotensin II on a high salt diet, and adrenal aldosterone release is more sensitive with restriction of sodium intake [6]. Because the term 'modulation' had been employed to describe such shifts in responsiveness in other endocrine systems, the inability of these individuals to change renal vascular and adrenal responsiveness to angiotensin II [7] was called 'nonmodulation' [8, 9] (fig. 1 and 2).

Several lines of evidence indicate that 'nonmodulation' is not part of a continuum, but rather represents a discrete subgroup present in about 45% of patients with normal renin and high renin essential hypertension [8, 9].

Sodium-Sensitive Hypertension

The frequent sensitivity of hypertension to sodium intake has long been recognized. In 1904, within a few years of the first recognition that hypertension represents a clinical disorder, Ambard and Beaujard [10] proposed that the increase in blood pressure reflected a failure to adapt to an excess of salt in the diet. Not long thereafter, Allen [11] in the USA demonstrated that a severe reduction of salt in the diet was effective in reducing blood pressure in about 60% of patients with hypertension. Both the French group and Allen believed that hypertension reflected an unknown renal defect that limited the individual's inability to handle salt. Since that time, confirmation of the frequency of sodium-sensitive hypertension has come from estimates based on sodium intake as therapy [12], the frequency of response to diuretics [13], and careful metabolic balance studies [14, 15] have confirmed a frequency of about 50–60%. The metabolic balance studies failed to identify a mechanism responsible for the blood pressure rise, but

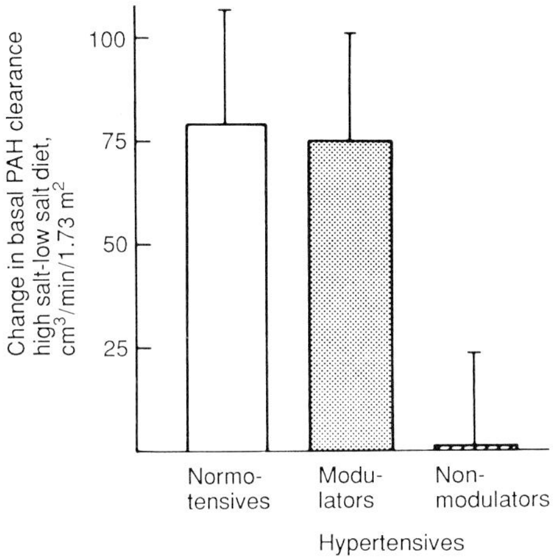

Fig. 1. Change in renal plasma flow on a shift from a high salt to a low salt diet. Note the similarity in the 20% change in renal plasma flow in normal subjects and in hypertensives with intact modulation and the absence of a change in renal plasma flow in the non-modulators. Figure from Redgrave et al. [18], with permission.

did demonstrate that individuals with salt-sensitive hypertension showed more positive sodium balance and gained more weight as their blood pressure rose [14, 15].

An abnormality involving the renal blood supply and adrenal aldosterone release, both crucial for sodium handling, raised the intriguing possibility to us that the unidentified patients in the metabolic balance studies were the nonmodulators. Indeed, that has turned out to be the case. Whether the pattern by which external sodium balance is achieved when sodium intake is restricted [16] or the acute response to a saline load [17] is employed as the index, nonmodulators show a clear inability to handle sodium. When the earlier metabolic balance study was replicated in a study in which external balance was first achieved on a restricted and then high salt intake, the nonmodulators showed more positive sodium balance as they gained more weight [16]; all of the sodium-sensitive hypertension that was identified occurred in that group [18].

Control of the Renal Circulation

In addition to blunted renal vascular responses to angiotensin II, two other abnormalities in the control of the renal circulation occur in nonmodulators that are germane both to renal vascular responses to angiotensin II

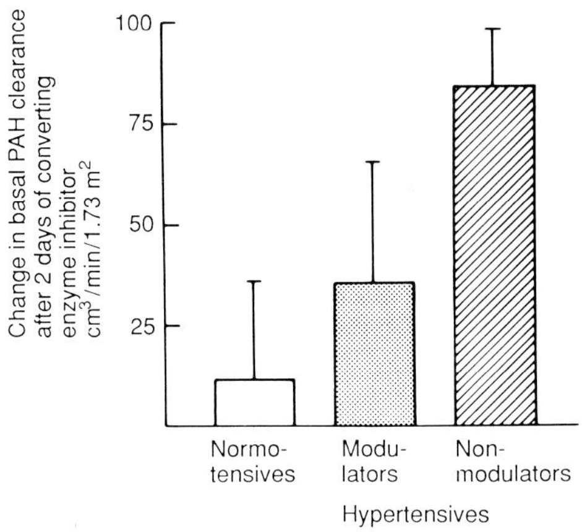

Fig. 2. Change in renal plasma flow after 2 days of converting enzyme inhibition in the same patients shown in figure 1. The study was performed on a high sodium intake so that the absence of a change in the normotensive subjects was anticipated. Note that the increase in renal plasma flow in non-modulators is essentially identical to the change in renal plasma flow with a shift in sodium intake. Figure from Redgrave et al. [18], with permission.

and to renal sodium handling. Normal individuals display parallel changes in renal blood flow as they change salt intake: in a shift from a high sodium to a low sodium intake renal blood flow falls, and rises with an increase in salt intake [3, 7, 9]. Patients with essential hypertension who have intact modulation show similar changes, but renal blood flow is fixed with shifts in sodium intake in nonmodulators [3, 7, 9, 16–18]. Again, this abnormality is not part of a continuum, but rather reflects a discrete limitation reflected in a bimodal distribution [16]. To the extent that intrarenal physical forces and filtration fraction contribute to the ability of the kidney to handle sodium, the limited renal vascular response to changes in sodium intake could account for the limited capacity of the kidney to handle sodium – described above.

A fixed renal blood supply in response to a physiological stimulus could reflect fixed, organic disease so common as a by-product of hypertension. On the other hand, multiple lines of evidence suggest that in some patients there is a functional abnormality of the renal blood supply, vasoconstriction, that contributes to the reduced renal blood flow [9]. ACE inhibition, long recognized as inducing a potentiated renal vasodilatation in essential hypertension [19, 20], is now recognized as producing preferential renal vasodilatation in the nonmodulator. Indeed, only nonmodulators display renal vasodilatation when an ACE inhibitor is administered on a high salt diet, when the renin system is suppressed [18].

ACE inhibition also restores renal vascular responsiveness to angiotensin II [18] and the capacity of the kidney to handle a sodium load [17]. We believe that the restoration of the ability of the kidney to handle a sodium load represents a major factor by which ACE inhibitors are effective at achieving goal blood pressure in patients with essential hypertension who are enjoying a typical high salt diet, and thus have a suppressed circulating renin-angiotensin system.

The restoration of the renal vascular response to angiotensin II following ACE inhibition also provides insight into mechanisms. If the renal vasodilatation reflected the accumulation of bradykinin because of reduced degradation, or prostaglandin release, the renal vasodilator response to ACE inhibition should have been associated with further blunting of renal vascular responsiveness to angiotensin II, since both prostaglandins and kinins share this characteristic [21].

Renin Release and Nonmodulation

Patients with nonmodulation at the steady state have either a normal or elevated level of plasma renin activity [5–7, 9], but two abnormalities of renin release have been identified in nonmodulators. In normal subjects on a low salt diet, intravenous infusion of saline rapidly reduces plasma renin activity and plasma aldosterone concentration, but only about 50% of the patients with essential hypertension show this rapid fall [22]. The same patients that had a blunted renin response also had a reduced rate of sodium excretion, and a transient pressor response to the saline infusion. These observations suggested the possibility that nonmodulation was involved. Indeed, subsequent studies showed that it is the nonmodulator that shows the delayed response to saline [23].

Saline-induced suppression of the renin-angiotensin system in the normal subjects did not involve simple plasma volume expansion, since the infusion of dextran in a volume to produce similar or more plasma volume expansion produced a delayed fall in plasma renin activity and plasma aldosterone concentration [22]. This observation made it possible to divide the stimulus into a 'sodium-sensitive' and a 'volume-sensitive' element. The rate of fall of plasma renin activity in response to saline in nonmodulators is identical to the normal response to dextran, the volume-sensitive signal. One attractive, but speculative interpretation of these data is that nonmodulators have a normal volume-sensing system, but lack the ability to respond to the specific signal emitted by sodium.

A second evidence of disregulation of renin release involves the so-called 'short feedback loop', by which angiotensin II reduces renin release. The response occurs within minutes, as opposed to the 'long feedback loop', which involves aldosterone release and sodium retention. Patients with essential hypertension frequently do not show renin suppression with angiotensin II infusion [24], an abnormality once again corrected by converting enzyme inhibition [25]. Again, after identification of the nonmodulating group, this abnormality was found to occur only in the nonmodulator [26].

Genetic Factors

A contribution of heredity to hypertension in many patients has long been recognized, but the precise factors inherited have been remarkably elusive. Information from renal transplantation, both in inbred animal models [27–29] and in man [30, 31] has suggested that the genetic information, at least some of the time, is coded in the kidney. Four lines of investigation have suggested that nonmodulation is inherited.

The first clue came from the frequency of a family history of hypertension in the parents of nonmodulators [16]. In the neighborhood of 90% of the nonmodulators in two studies have a parent with hypertension, where the family history could be evaluated, as opposed to a rate of about 30% in essential hypertensives in whom modulation was intact. The second line of investigation involves the identification of features identical to nonmodulation in the offspring of hypertensives, involving both the adrenal gland and the kidney. In the adrenal, plasma aldosterone concentration in the offspring of hypertensives studied on a low salt diet was substantially lower than the concentration in the offspring of normotensive parents, despite a similar level of plasma renin activity and plasma angiotensin II concentration [32]. In an elegant study of aldosterone release in response to angiotensin II infusion performed by Beretta-Picolli et al. [33], aldosterone release was shown to be blunted in the offspring of hypertensives but not normotensive parents [34]. This study was especially impressive because it was performed in Japan, where an ad libitum intake is especially rich in sodium chloride. We have confirmed that observation restrospectively in data for our earlier studies, and prospectively, the calcium channel blocking agent, diltiazem, increased renal blood flow, preferentially in 50% of the offspring of hypertensives, but not in the control group made up of the normotensive offspring of normotensive parents [32]. Diltiazem blocked the action of angiotensin II on the renal blood supply in that study. The specificity of that response was confirmed by the observation that no difference could be identified in the renal vascular response to the vasodilator acetylcholine as a function of family history.

A third line of evidence involves red blood cells sodium:lithium countertransport. Lithium countertransport is increased not only in many hypertensives, but also in their normotensive offspring [35–37]. There is a striking increase in the frequency with which increased lithium countertransport occurs in nonmodulation [38, 39]. Unfortunately, because of the number of confounding variables that influence lithium countertransport, that determination will be useful in identifying nonmodulators only at the extremes of countertransport.

Finally, in a study still in progress involving multiple family members, renal plasma flow and its response to angiotensin have been found in aggregate significantly in the nonmodulator [16, 17]. There is evidence that sodium handling also is influenced by heredity, and is modified by a family history of hypertension [40]. It will be intriguing to ascertain whether that genetic influence expressed itself through nonmodulation.

Eqully, speculative, and equally intriguing, is the possibility that nonmodulation has implications for the pathogenesis of renal disease. About one-third of patients with type I diabetes mellitus will develop nephropathy, and two thirds will not, despite an apparently identical severity and duration of disease. Studies in animal models have suggested a powerful role for renal hemodynamic factors, but have not provided an explanation for the fact that 100% of rats but only 33% of people will progress to nephropathy. The information to indicate that the control of the renal circulation is altered not only in nonmodulators, but also in their normotensive offspring, may be relevant. Patients with diabetes mellitus at risk of nephropathy display elevated red blood cell sodium:lithium countertransport and a striking family history of hypertension [41, 42], features that they share with nonmodulation. To the extent that nonmodulators and their normotensive offspring act as though they have elevated intrarenal angiotensin II concentration – reflected in a blunted renal vascular response to angiotensin II, blunted renin release in response to saline and angiotensin II, and a potentiated renal vascular response to converting enzyme inhibition – the metabolic disarray of diabetes mellitus superimposed on a disordered control of the renal circulation could lead to glomerular hypertension and its consequences.

Implications for Nuclear Medicine

The captopril test for renovascular hypertension is rapidly becoming a standard [43, 44] as attested to by several elements in this monograph. Because of the much greater prevalence of essential hypertension, most tests are performed in patients with essential hypertension, and provide nothing beyond ruling out a renovascular process. If the test can be modified to identify the nonmodulator – renal vasodilatation following captopril despite a high salt diet – the information yield would be enhanced substantially. Why identify them? They have a predictable therapeutic response [18].

References

1 Dahl LK: Metabolic aspects of hypertension. Annu Rev Med 1963;14:69–93.
2 Gutman RA, Forrey AW, Flet WP, et al: Vasopressor-induced natriuresis and altered intrarenal hemodynamics in cirrhotic man. Clin Sci Mol Med 1973;45:19–34.
3 Hollenberg NK, Merrill JP: Intrarenal perfusion in the young essential hypertensive: A subpopulation resistant to sodium restriction. Trans Assoc Am (Physicians) 1970;83:93–101.
4 Williams GH, Rose LI, Dluhy RG, et al: Abnormal responsiveness of the renin aldosterone system to acute stimulation in patients with essential hypertension. Ann Intern Med 1970;72:317–326.
5 Williams GH, Tuck ML, Sullivan JM, et al: Parallel adrenal and renal abnormalities in the young patient with essential hypertension. Am J Med 1982;72:907–914.
6 Hollenberg NK, Chenitz WR, Adams DF, et al: Reciprocal influence of salt intake on adrenal glomerulosa and renal vascular responses to angiotensin II in normal man. J Clin Invest 1970;54:34–42.
7 Shoback DM, Williams GH, Hollenberg NK, et al: Endogenous angiontensin II as a determinant of sodium modulated changes in tissue responsiveness to angiotensin II in normal man. J Clin Endocrinol Metab 1983;57:764–770.
8 Williams GH, Hollenberg NK: Abnormal adrenal and renal responses to angiotensin II in essential hypertension: Implications for pathogenesis; in Carey RM (ed): Clinical Endocrinology: Is Essential Hypertension an Endocrine Disease? London, Butterworth, 1985, vol 7, pp 184–211.
9 Hollenberg NK, Williams GH: Sensitivity to sodium and nonmodulation of renal and adrenal responsiveness to angiotensin II. Implications for the pathogenesis of hypertension; in Zanchetti A, Tarazi RC (eds.): Handbook of Hypertension. New York, Elsevier, 1986, vol 8, chapt 25, pp 520–522.
10 Ambard L, Beaujard E: Causes de l'hypertension arterielle. Arch Intern Med 1904;1:520–533.
11 Allen FM: Treatment of Kidney Disease and High Blood Pressure. Morristown, The Psychiatric Institute, 1925, p 206.
12 Chapman B: Some effects of the rice-fruit diet in patients with essential hypertension; in Bell ET (ed): Hypertension: A Symposium, Minneapolis 1951, pp 504–516.
13 Freis E: Comparative effects of tierynafen and hydrochlorothiazide in the treatment of hypertension (Veterans Adminstration Cooperative Study Group on Antihypertensive Agents). N Engl J Med 1979;301:293–297.
14 Kawasaki T, Delea CS, Bartter FC, et al: The effect of high sodium and low sodium intakes on blood pressure and other related variables in human subjects with idiopathic hypertension. Am J Med 1978;64:193–198.
15 Fujita T, Henry WL, Bartter FC, et al: Factors influencing blood pressure in salt-sensitive patients with hypertension. Am J Med 1980;69:334–344.

16 Hollenberg NK, Williams GH: Abnormal renal sodium handling in essential hypertension: Relation to failure to renal and adrenal modulation of responses to angiotensin II. Am J Med 1986;81:412–418.
17 Rystedt LL, Williams GH, Hollenberg NK: The renal and endocrine response to saline infusion in essential hypertension. Hypertension 1986;8:217–222.
18 Redgrave JE, Rabinowe SL, Hollenberg NK, et al: Correction of abnormal renal blood flow response to angiotensin II by converting enzyme inhibition in essential hypertensives. J Clin Invest 1985;75:1285–1290.
19 Williams GH, Hollenberg NK: Accentuated vascular and endocrine responses to SQ 20881 in hypertension. N Engl J Med 1977;297:184–188.
20 Hollenberg NK, Meggs LG, Williams GH, et al: Sodium intake and renal responses to captopril in normal man and in essential hypertension. Kidney 1981;20:240–245.
21 Meggs LG, Katzberg RW, DeLeeuw P, et al: Specific desensitization of the canine renal vasculature to angiotensin II despite cycloxygenase inhibition. Yale J Biol Med 1985;58:453–458.
22 Tuck ML, Williams GH, Dluhy RG, et al: A delayed suppression of the renin-aldosterone axis following saline infusion in human hypertension. Circ Res 1976;39:711–716.
23 Rabinowe SL, Redgrave JE, Rysedt LL, et al: Renin suppression by saline is blunted in non-modulating essential hypertension. Hypertension 1987;10:404–408.
24 Dluhy RG, Bavli SZ, Leung FK, et al: Abnormal adrenal responsiveness and angiotensin II dependency in high renin essential hypertension. J Clin Invest 1979;64:1270–1276.
25 LeBoff MS, Dluhy RG, Hollenberg NK, et al: Abnormal renin short feedback loop in essential hypertension is reversible with converting enzyme inhibition. J Clin Invest 1982;70:335–341.
26 Seely EW, Moore TJ, Rogacz S, et al: Abnormal angiotensin II suppression of plasma renin activity in non-modulators is corrected with converting enzyme inhibition. Abstract from the American Heart Association's 41st Annual Fall Conference and Scientific Sessions, New Orleans 1987.
27 Bianchi G, Fox U, DiFrancesco GF, et al: Blood pressure changes produced by kidney cross-transplantation between spontaneously hypertensive rats (SHR) and normotensive rats (NR). Clin Sci Mol Med 1974;47:435.
28 Dahl LK, Heine M: Primary role of renal hemografts in setting blood pressure levels in rats. Circ Res 1975;36:692.
29 Kawabe K, Watanabe TX, Shiono K, et al: Influence of blood pressure of renal isografts between spontaneously hypertensive and normotensive rats utilizing the F_1 hybrids. Jap Heart J 1978;19:886.
30 Guidi E, Bianchi G, Dallosia V, et al: Influence of familial hypertension of the donor on the blood pressure and antihypertensive therapy of kidney graft recipients. Nephron 1982;30:318.
31 Curtis JJ, Luke RG, Dustan HP, et al: Remission of essential hypertension after renal transplantation. N Engl J Med 1983;309:1009.
32 Blackshear JL, Garnic D, Williams GH, et al: Exaggerated renal vascular response to calcium entry blockade in first-degree relatives of essential hypertensives: Possible role of intrarenal angiotensin II. Hypertension 1987;9:384–389.
33 Beretta-Picolli C, Pusterla C, Stadler P, et al: Blunted aldosterone responsiveness to AII in normotensive subjects with familial predisposition to essential hypertension. J Hypertens 1988;61:57–61.
34 Uneda S, Fukishima S, Fujika Y, et al: Renal hemodynamics and renin angiotensin system in adolescents genetically predisposed to essential hypertension. J Hypertens 1986; 2(suppl 3): 437–439.

35 Canessa M, Adranga N, Solomon H, et al: Increased sodium-lithium countertransport in red cells of patients with essential hypertension. N Engl J Med 1980;302:772–776.
36 Cooper R, Miller T, Trevisan M, et al: Family history of hypertension and red cell cation transport in high school students. J Hypertens 1983;1:145–152.
37 Clegg G, Morgan DB, Davidson C: The heterogenicity of essential hypertension: Relation between lithium efflux and sodium content of erythrocytes and a family history of hypertension. Lancet 1982;ii:891–894.
38 Redgrave JE, Canessa M, Gleason R, Hollenberg NK, Williams GH: Red blood cell lithium: sodium countertransport in non-modulating essential hypertension. Hypertension 1989;13:721–726.
39 Dluhy RG, Hopkins P, Hollenberg NK, et al: Heritable abnormalities of the renin-angiotensin-aldosterone system in essential hypertension. J Cardiovasc Pharmacol 1988;12(3):149–154.
40 Luft FC, Rankin LI, Bloch R, et al: Cardiovascular and humoral responses to extremes of sodium intake in normal black and white men. Circulation 1979;60:697–703.
41 Krolewski AS, Canessa M, Warram JH, et al: Predisposition to hypertension and susceptibility to renal disease in insulin-dependent diabetes mellitus. N Engl J Med 1988;318:140–145.
42 Mangill R, Bending JJ, Scott G, et al: Increased sodium-lithium countertransport activity in red cells of patients with insulin-dependent diabetes and nephropathy. N Engl J Med 1988;318:146–150.
43 Sfakianakis GN, Sfakianakis E, Bourgoignie J: Renal scintigraphy following angiotensin-converting enzyme inhibition in the diagnosis of renovascular hypertension (captopril scintigraphy); in Freeman LM, Weissman HS (eds): Nuclear Medicine Annual 1988. New York, Raven Press, 1988, pp 125–170.
44 Wilcox CS, Williams CM, Smith TB, et al: Diagnostic uses of angiotensin converting enzyme inhibitors in renovascular hypertension. Am J Hypertens 1988:344S–349S.

Norman K. Hollenberg, MD, PhD, Departments of Medicine and Radiology, Brigham and Women's Hospital, 75 Francis Street, Boston, MA 02115 (USA)

Blaufox MD, Hollenberg NK, Raynaud C (eds): Radionuclides in Nephro-Urology.
Contrib Nephrol. Basel, Karger, 1990, vol 79, pp 11–16

^{99m}Tc-MAG$_3$: Chemistry and Biokinetics of By-Products

W. Brandau[a], *B. Bubeck*[b], *O. Schober*[a], *E. Weber*[c], *D.M. Taylor*[d]

[a]Department of Nuclear Medicine, University of Münster; [b]Department of Nuclear Medicine, University of Heidelberg; [c]German Cancer Research Center, Heidelberg; [d]Institute of Radiation Toxicology, University of Heidelberg, FRG

During the last few years a number of ^{99m}Tc complexes have been developed and discussed as potential replacements of radioiodinated *o*-hippuric acid (OIH) in renal function studies. However, none of these complexes showed a biological behavior similar, or superior, to that of OIH. In 1985, a ^{99m}Tc-complex containing a N_3S core, technetium-99m-mercaptoacetylglycylglycylglycine (^{99m}Tc-MAG$_3$), was described by Fritzberg et al. [1] which showed biokinetic data close to that of OIH. Already the first clinical studies indicated that ^{99m}Tc-MAG$_3$ is a useful radiopharmaceutical for the substitution of OIH in renal function studies [2, 3]. Nevertheless, some problems occurred with the 'kit-formulation', which is essential for wide clinical use of this radiopharmaceutical. The subject of our work is the biological investigation of ^{99m}Tc-MAG$_3$ and of the by-products occurring during the labeling reaction.

Materials and Methods

The precursor of MAG$_3$ was prepared starting with the synthesis of S-benzoylthioglycolic acid. The subsequent condensation with N-hydroxysuccinimide led to succinimidyl-S-benzoylthioglycolate, an active storable ester [4]. Aminolysis of this compound with glycylglycylglycine gave S-benzoyl-mercaptoacetylglycylglyclyglycine (S-Bz-MAG$_3$) in an overall yield of 42% [5]. ^{1}H-NMR (500 MHz, DMSO-d$_6$): 3.72 ppm (d, 2H), (–N–C$\underline{H}_2$–CO–), 3.75 ppm (d, 2H), (–N–C$\underline{H}_2$–CO–), 3.79 ppm (d, 2H), (–N–C$\underline{H}_2$–CO–), 3.89 ppm (s, 2H), (–S–C$\underline{H}_2$–CO–), 7.55–7.95 ppm (m, 5H), (aromatic), 8.05 ppm (t, 1H), (–CO–N$\underline{H}$–CH$_2$–), 8.19 ppm (t, 1H), (–CO–N$\underline{H}$–CH$_2$–), 8.4 ppm (t, 1H), (–CO–N$\underline{H}$–CH$_2$–). Elemental analysis: Calculated for $C_{15}H_{17}N_3O_6S$: C, 49.04%; H, 4.66%; N, 11.44%; S, 8.73%; Found: C, 48.65%; H, 5.13%; N, 12.60%; S, 7.55%.

Labeling Procedure

A 'kit preparation', containing potassium gluconate, S-Bz-MAG_3 and stannous chloride, was used. In contrast to the procedure published by Fritzberg et al. [6], we used only 0.5 mg of the precursor and 15 µg stannous chloride to prepare one kit. Labeling yields were determined during HPLC purification. All fractions were collected, adjusted to a defined volume and monitored in a dose calibrator.

Commerical kits were labeled as specified by the distributor (Mallinckrodt, Petten, The Netherlands) and were analyzed by means of HPLC. HPLC separations were performed with an isocratic system (Latek, Eppelheim, FRG) using reversed phase columns (250 × 4.6 mm, Nucleosil, C_{18}, 5 µm; Macherey & Nagel, Düren, FRG). The columns were eluted at a flow rate of 1 ml/min with 10% of ethanol in 0.05 *M* phosphate buffer at pH = 7.0.

Electrophoreses (120 V, 70 min) were performed on cellulose acetate strips at various pH values between 4.0 and 7.4.

Animal Studies

The scintigraphic studies were performed with female Sprague-Dawley rats (180–200 g). The animals were anesthetized by intraperitoneal injection of chloral hydrate (500 mg/kg) 30 min prior to the beginning of the study. Each animal was positioned in a supine position and placed in an exactly defined distance under the camera, which was fitted with a pinhole collimator. After the injection of the respective technetium compound (2.7–8.2 MBq, 0.3–0.8 ml) into a lateral tail vein, 30 images were recorded in 1-min intervals. Regions of interest (ROI) were placed over the liver, the kidneys and the urinary bladder. The counts/ROI were corrected for physical decay of ^{99m}Tc, tissue absorption and for geometric factors of the collimator. Details of this correction procedure and the validation of the method are described elsewhere [7]. From these data, time activity curves were calculated for each ROI.

Patient Studies

Steady-state clearance data of ^{131}I-OIH and ^{99m}Tc-MAG_3 were determined in 124 patients simultaneously by a special feedback-controlled infusion pump device [8, 9]. Protein binding was determined by ultrafiltration.

Results

Chemistry

The benzoyl-protected precursor of mercaptoacetylglycylglycylglycine was synthesized following the synthetic route published previously [5]. The overall yield is somewhat lower than in the synthesis published by Fritzberg et al. [6]. The advantage of the procedure described here is that succinimidyl-S-benzoylthioglycolate is a storable active ester [4], which can be coupled with various oligopeptides. This offers the possibility of synthesizing modified N_3S ligands in a simple one-step reaction. More than 400 own kit preparations gave ^{99m}Tc-MAG_3 in radiochemical yields of 84–97%.

Within one batch the radiochemical yield is highly reproducible; only minor differences of about 4% could be observed. Figure 1 depicts typical HPLC chromatograms of two ^{99m}Tc-MAG_3 preparations. Although the labeling yield of the commercial preparation is somewhat higher, the

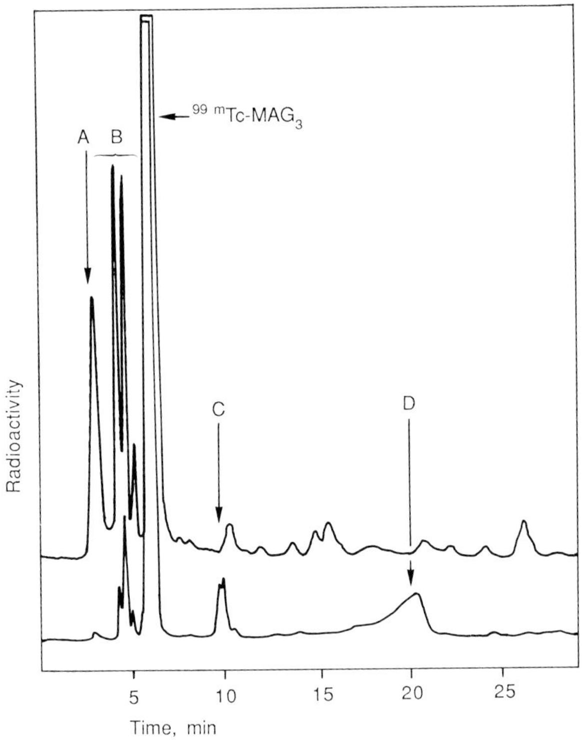

Fig. 1. HPLC profiles of $^{99m}Tc-MAG_3$. Top: commercial product radiochemical yield: 95%; bottom: own product radiochemical yield: 92%. Stationary phase: Nucleosil 5-C_{18}, 250 × 4.6 mm; mobile phase: 10% ethanol in 0.05 *M* phosphate buffer (pH = 7.0); flow rate: 1 ml/min.

by-products are essentially the same. In all preparations 'A' and 'B' were the main impurities. Neither, 'reduced hydrolyzed technetium' nor free pertechnetate could be detected. In commercial kits (n = 11) the radiochemical yield was determined to be 92%, including two preparations with 78% and 87% initial yield.

The time-dependent stability of the kits is excellent. Up to 6 months at −18 °C no changes in the labeling yield could be observed. Furthermore, the preparations appeared not to be sensitive to the source of technetium or to the amount of pertechnetate added (up to 16 GBq).

Electrophoreses at pH 4.0–7.4 revealed that $^{99m}Tc-MAG_3$ is negatively charged in this pH range. These results are in agreement with the octanol/water partition coefficients which were determined to be between 0.7×10^3 at pH = 7.4 and 6.5×10^2 at pH = 4.0.

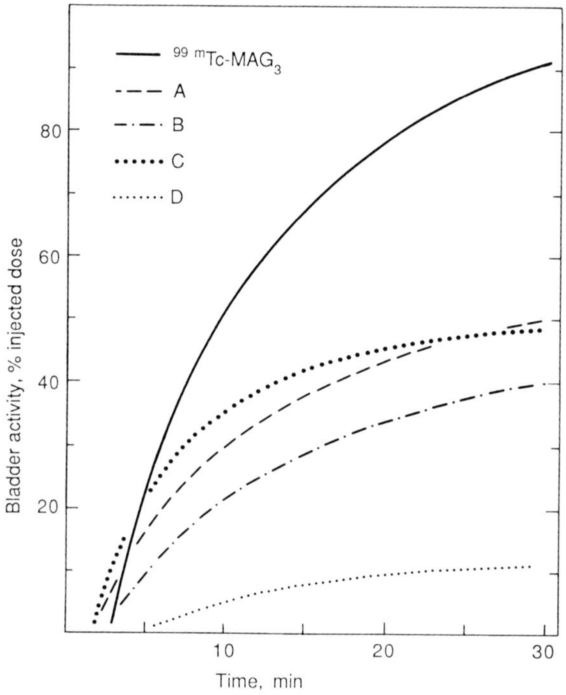

Fig. 2. Cumulative excretion of ^{99m}Tc-MAG$_3$ and the impurities A, B, C and D into the urinary bladder of rats.

Biology

Figure 2 shows the cumulative excretion of ^{99m}Tc-MAG$_3$ and of the by-products into the urinary bladder of rats. As is obvious, only ^{99m}Tc-MAG$_3$ is excreted in a sufficient high degree into the urinary bladder within 30 min. This result corresponds with the renograms obtained from rats [5] which show that the compounds 'B' and 'D' are not significantly eliminated by the kidneys during the period of investigation. The compounds 'B', 'C' and 'D' were excreted in such a high degree through the hepatobiliary route that they would spoil quantitative renal function studies if they were present in significant amounts.

Patient Studies

The plasma protein binding of ^{99m}Tc-MAG$_3$ has been determined to be 90% and is significantly higher than that of *o*-iodohippuric acid (74%). These data implicate that the glomerular filtrated fraction of ^{99m}Tc-MAG$_3$ is negligible and its clearance corresponds with the tubular extraction rate

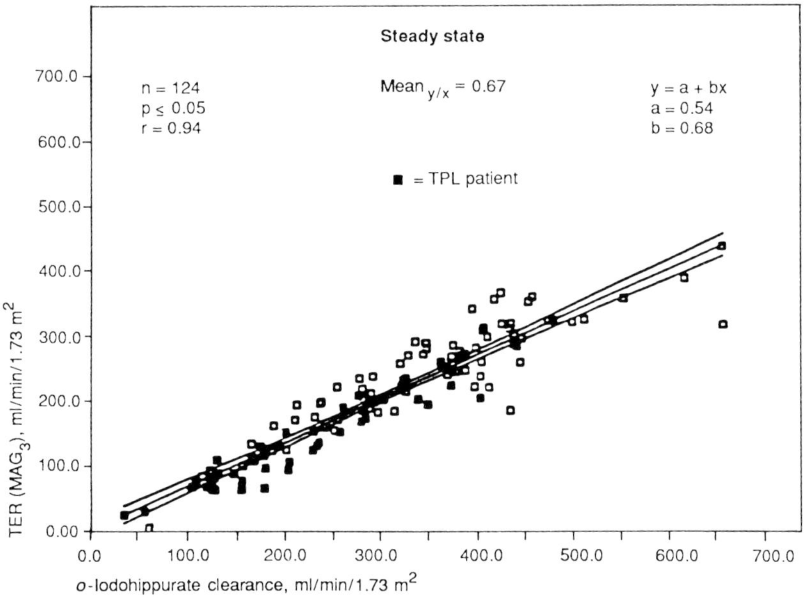

Fig. 3. Simultaneously determined clearances of HPLC-purified ^{99m}Tc-MAG$_3$ and ^{131}I-OIH under steady-state conditions.

(TER) of this compound. Figure 3 shows the results of 124 simultaneous clearance measurements with ^{131}I-OIH and HPLC-purified ^{99m}Tc-MAG$_3$. The TER (MAG$_3$) was determined to be 67% of the OIH clearance. This value was found to be identical under steady-state conditions as well as under slope conditions. The correlation coefficient of 0.94 indicates that ^{99m}Tc-MAG$_3$ is an adequate alternative to OIH in quantitative renal function studies.

Discussion

We conclude that the impurities indicated as 'A', 'B', 'C' and 'D' must be excluded from ^{99m}Tc-MAG$_3$ preparations because of their low renal elimination. The renal clearance of HPLC-purified ^{99m}Tc-MAG$_3$, which is described as the TER of this compound, is only 67% of that of OIH in humans [8,9]. In our opinion, this ratio would be unfavorably influenced by the presence of by-products. The results from our animal experiments and human studies reveal that the observations made by other authors, especially the visualization of the gallbladder in humans [10, 11, 12], is more a problem of the radiochemical purity of the preparation than of the biological behavior of $^{99m}Tc-MAG_3$ itself. HPLC-purified $^{99m}Tc-MAG_3$ is not extrarenally eliminated in measurable amounts and no visualization of the gallbladder could be observed.

^{99m}Tc-mercaptoacetylglycylglyclyglycine is a very useful radiopharmaceutical for renal function studies, having all the advantages of the radionuclide ^{99m}Tc. Nevertheless, the radiochemical yield of the preparation should be carefully inspected to prevent pitfalls which are caused by the presence of radioactive by-products.

References

1 Fritzberg AR, Kasina S, Johnson DL, et al: Triamide mercaptide (N_3S) ligands for Tc-99m as potential Tc-99m renal function agents (abstract). J Nucl Med 1985;26:19.

2 Bubeck B, Brandau W, Dreikorn K, et al: Clinical comparison of I-131 o-Iodohippurate with Tc-99m CO_2-DADS-A an Tc-99m MAG_3 by simultaneous double tracer measurement. NucCompact 1986;17:135.

3 Taylor A, Eshima D, Fritzberg AR, et al: Comparison of Iodine-131 OIH and Technetium-99m MAG_3 renal imaging in volunteers. J Nucl Med 1986;27:795.

4 Schneider RF, Subramanian G, Field TA, et al: N, N'-bis (S-benzoylmercaptoacetamido) ethylenediamine and propylenediamine ligands as renal function imaging agents. I. Alternate synthetic methods. J Nucl Med 1984;25:233.

5 Brandau W, Bubeck B, Eisenhut M, et al: Technetium-99m-labeled renal function and imaging agents. III. Synthesis of $^{99m}Tc-MAG_3$ and biodistribution of by-products. Appl Radiat Isot 1988;39:121.

6 Fritzberg AR, Kasina S, Eshima D, et al: Synthesis and biological evaluation of technetium-99m-MAG_3 as a hippuran replacement. J Nucl Med 1986;27:111.

7 Brandau W: Physikalisch-chemische und biologische Eigenschaften von Technetium-99m-Amin-Komplexen; Dissertation, University of Heidelberg 1985.

8 Bubeck B, Brandau W, Weidenhammer K, et al: The tubular extraction rate of Tc-99m-MAG_3: a new quantitative parameter of renal function. Nuc Compact 1987;18:260.

9 Bubeck B, Brandau W, Steinbächer M, et al: Technetium-99m-labeled renal function and imaging agents. II. Clinical evaluation of $^{99m}Tc-MAG_3$ (^{99m}Tc-mercaptoacetylglycylglycylglycine). Nucl Med Biol 1988;15:109.

10 Taylor A, Eshima D, Christian P, et al: Tc-99m MAG_3 kit formulation: Preliminary results in normal volunteers and patients with renal failure. J Nucl Med 1988;29:616.

11 Jafri RA, Britton KE, Nimmon CC, et al: Technetium-99m MAG_3, a comparison with Iodine-123 and Iodine-131 Orthoiodohippurate, in patients with renal disorders, J Nucl Med 1988;29:147.

12 Coveney JR, Robbins MS: Comparison of technetium-99m MAG_3 kit with HPLC-purified technetium-99m MAG_3 an OIH in Rats. J Nucl Med 1987;28:1881.

Dr. Wolfgang Brandau, Westfälische Wilhelms-Universität Münster,
Klinik und Poliklinik für Nuklearmedizin, Albert-Schweitzer-Strasse 33,
D-4400 Münster (FRG)

Blaufox MD, Hollenberg NK, Raynaud C (eds): Radionuclides in Nephro-Urology.
Contrib Nephrol. Basel, Karger, 1990, vol 79, pp 17–20

Handling of ^{99m}Tc-MAG$_3$ in the Kidney

Charlotte Müller-Suur, Roland Müller-Suur

Department of Physiology and Medical Physics, Uppsala University, Uppsala, and Department of Clinical Physiology, Karolinska Institute, Danderyds Hospital, Stockholm, Sweden

Recently a new promising renal imaging radiopharmaceutical ^{99m}Tc-mercaptoacetyltriglycine (MAG$_3$), has been introduced [1] and been studied both in clinical trials [2–5] as well as animal experiments [6, 7]. The similarity between MAG$_3$ and hippurate has been outlined by most of the authors and MAG$_3$ thus been recommended as a substitute for hippurate in renal function studies. However, several differences between these two substances have also been reported [6, 7] and the present study was performed to further characterize the renal excretion mechanism for MAG$_3$ in comparison with hippurate. In the present study, a micropuncture technique was applied in rats on surface glomeruli for direct measurement of glomerular filtration of MAG$_3$ and on proximal and distal tubules to outline its secretory capacity along the nephron. Plasma protein binding measurements together with whole kidney clearances were also used to estimate the filtered and secreted part of the total excretion of MAG$_3$ in comparison with hippurate.

Methods

Male Wistar rats (body weights between 180 and 300 g) of a special strain with surface glomeruli were anesthetized and prepared for micropuncture as described earlier [8]. The left kidney was prepared free and placed in a lucite chamber, fixed with cotton tissue and the surface illuminated. The jugular and the femoral vein were also cannulated for infusion of radionuclide solutions together with Ringer's solution to give a total infusion rate of 1 ml/h·100 g b.w. ^{99m}Tc-MAG$_3$ (kit prepared, Mallinckrodt, Petten, The Netherlands) and ^{125}I-hippurate (Amersham International Hants, UK) were diluted in the final solution to give approximately 18 and 2.7 MBq/h, respectively. In two separate rats, ^{3}H-inulin (Amersham) was infused at a rate of 2.7 MBq/h solely.

Surface glomeruli appearing as capillary balls at the surface of the kidney were punctured with sharpened glass pipets of 5–7 µm outer diameter. After injection of an oil block into the proximal tubule the ultrafiltrate from Bowman's space was collected. Late proximal tubules and early distal tubules were also micropunctured and the tubular fluid sampled in a similar way. The radioactivity of the microsamples was counted in a well-type counter. The ^{99m}Tc activity was counted the same day and the samples were recounted after the decay of ^{99m}Tc for their ^{125}I activity. ^{3}H-inulin activity was counted after diluting the samples with scintillation cocktail in a scintillation counter. The volume of the samples was measured in precalibrated parallel-bore capillaries. Corresponding plasma samples were taken immediately after each puncture and timed final urine samples were also taken and analyzed.

For measurement of plasma protein binding of MAG_3 and hippurate, arterial plasma was centrifuged in special vials (Centrifree; Amicon, Mass., USA) at 3,000 *g*. Radioactivity of plasma before centifugation and of the ultrafiltrate gave the amount of protein binding.

For whole kidney clearance measurements with simultaneous determinations of GFR, 6 separate rats were used with the same animal preparation as above. Both ^{99m}Tc-MAG_3 (1.8 MBq/h) and ^{125}I-hippurate (360 KBq/h) and ^{51}Cr-EDTA (320 KBq/h) were infused simultaneously at a rate of 1 ml/h·100 g b.w. Plasma and urine aliquots were measured for their radioactivity in a well-type gammacounter with background, cross talk and decay correction. MAG_3 and hippurate clearance and GFR, i.e. EDTA clearance, were calculated in the usual manner, corrected for kidney wet weight. The amount of filtrated and secreted MAG_3 or hippurate could be calculated from the protein-free tracer fraction times GFR and total clearance minus filtrated amount respectively.

Results and Discussion

Glomerular micropuncture showed in 18 glomeruli of 6 rats that the ratio of activity of ultrafiltrate in Bowan's space to that of the arterial plasma (UF/P) for MAG_3 was 0.24 ± 0.01 and for hippurate 0.64 ± 0.03 ($p < 0.001$). In seven glomeruli of 2 rats the UF/P inulin was 1.04 ± 0.04. This demonstrates that only 23% of MAG_3 in the arterial plasma is free filtrated, whereas 61% of hippurate and all inulin is free filtrated. In vitro measurements showed that MAG_3 was bound to proteins in rat plasma at $80 \pm 1.5\%$ as compared to $32 \pm 2\%$ for hippurate ($p < 0.001$).

Micropuncture of proximal and distal tubules showed that the tubular fluid to plasma ratio (TF/P) of MAG_3 was 2.68 ± 0.34 in proximal tubules ($n = 10$) whereas the TF/P of hippurate was 5.46 ± 0.71 ($p < 0.001$). The TF/P values for MAG_3 in the distal tubules was 13.7 ± 1.47 ($n = 8$) and 24.01 ± 3.36 for hippurate ($p < 0.01$). Thus in both cases the TF/P values for MAG_3 were lower than those of hippurate. The same is true in the final urine where the urine to plasma ratio (U/P) for MAG_3 was 584 ± 99 and for hippurate $1,094 \pm 261$ ($p < 0.05$).

In 6 separate rats the simultaneous measurements of both the glomerular filtration rate by ^{51}Cr-EDTA and the hippurate clearance and MAG_3 clearance showed 1.28 ± 0.05, 3.25 ± 0.08 and 2.27 ± 0.08 ml/min·g kidney weight, respectively. Thus the MAG_3 clearance was significantly lower than that of hippurate ($p < 0.001$). The amount of filtration calculated from GFR and the protein-free plasma fraction was 0.26 ± 0.01 ml/min·g kidney

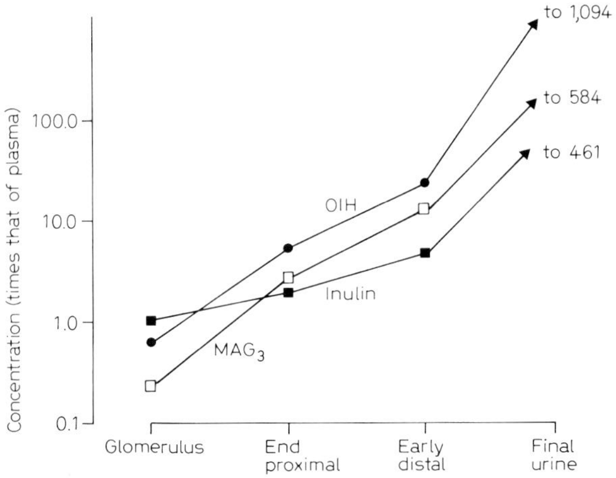

Fig. 1. Concentration profile of MAG$_3$, hippurate and inulin along the nephron. Observe logarithmic scale. Inulin data are from Müller-Suur et al. [8].

weight for MAG$_3$ and 0.87 ± 0.04 for hippurate ($p < 0.001$). The amount of secretion of MAG$_3$ and hippurate was 2.00 ± 0.10 and 2.39 ± 0.08 ml/min·g kidney weight ($p < 0.05$), respectively.

Already in earlier studies the similarity of MAG$_3$ to hippurate concerning its high renal clearance and the inhibitory effect of probenecid [1–5] led to the conclusion that the same transport mechanism may be involved for the two substances. The higher amount of MAG$_3$ bound to plasma proteins was taken as an argument for very low glomerular filtration. In all studies the renal clearance of MAG$_3$ was shown to be considerably less than that for hippurate. There is experimental evidence that the affinity of MAG$_3$ to rat tubules is less than that of hippurate [5, 6] and the present study adds more evidence to these observations. The present results demonstrate that the amount of MAG$_3$ in the glomerulus is less than that of inulin, only 23% of it, and also lower than that of hippurate. Since it correlates strongly with the amount of protein-free MAG$_3$ in arterial plasma the glomerular filtration barrier seems to permit all protein-free MAG$_3$ to be filtrated. Since high protein binding of MAG$_3$ has also been found in human plasma, restricted glomerular filtration will also exist in humans. The present findings further demonstrate a lower secretory capacity for MAG$_3$ than for hippurate along the entire nephron according to the lower TF/P and U/P ratio of MAG$_3$. Fitting the present data of MAG$_3$ and hippurate in a graph showing the concentration profile along the nephron (fig. 1), it becomes obvious that MAG$_3$ can be placed inbetween hippurate and inulin. The inulin data for proximal and distal tubules were taken from an earlier study of our laboratory [8] since for technical reasons we were not able to determine ^{3}H-inulin activity simultaneously with ^{125}I activity. Since the inulin concentration profile indicates the effect of water reabsorption along the nephron, a profile higher than that of inulin indicates net secretion both for MAG_3 and hippurate. Several possible factors may contribute to a lower secretion of MAG_3 than that of hippurate. Penetration of MAG_3 into blood cells was found to be low both in rats [7] and humans [4] compared to hippurate. The same may be true also for the penetration into tubular secretory cells and thus be responsible for lower outward transport capacities into the tubular lumen. The high protein binding of MAG_3 may also be involved in such a hypothetical chain of events. Furthermore, other unknown factors decreasing the affinity to the tubular cells may be involved and further experiments are necessary.

Summarizing, we have demonstrated that the lower clearance of MAG_3 is partly explained by a lower amount of filtration, due to a higher plasma protein binding, but also by a lower tubular secretion rate along the entire nephron.

References

1 Fritzberg AR, Kasina S, Eshima D, et al: Synthesis and biologic evaluation of technetium-99m-MAG_3 as a hippuran replacement. J Nucl Med 1986;27:111–116.
2 Taylor A, Ziffer JA, Stevens A, et al: Clinical comparison of ^{131}I-orthoiodohippurate and the kit formulation of ^{99m}Tc-mercaptoacetyltriglycine. Radiology 1989;170:721–725.
3 Al-Nahhas AA, Jafri RA, Britton KE, et al: Clinical experience with ^{99m}Tc-MAG_3, mercaptoacetyltriglycine, and a comparison with ^{99m}Tc-DTPA. Eur J Nucl Med 1988;14:453–462.
4 Müller-Suur R, Bois-Svensson I, Mesko L: A comparative study of renal scintigraphy and clearance with ^{99m}Tc-MAG_3 and ^{123}I-hippurate in patients with renal disorders. J Nucl Med, accepted for publication 1989.
5 Brandau W, Bubeck B, Berger J, et al: Excretion characteristics of ^{99m}Tc-MAG_3 in patients; in Schmidt HEA, Buraggi GL (eds): Nuclear Medicine, Stuttgart, Schattauer, 1989, pp 409–412.
6 Coveney JR, Pilcher GD, Robbins MS: ^{99m}Tc-MAG_3 and ^{131}I *o*-iodohippurate (OIH) transport kinetics in rat kidney slices. Eur J Nucl Med 1988;14:256.
7 Müller-Suur R, Müller-Suur C: Renal and extrarenal handling of a new imaging compound (^{99m}Tc-MAG_3) in the rat. Eur J Nucl Med 1986;12:438–442.
8 Müller-Suur R, Norlen BJ, Persson AEG: Resetting of tubuloglomerular feedback in rat kidneys after unilateral nephrectomy. Kidney Int 1980;18:48–57.

Roland Müller-Suur, MD, Karolinska Institute, Department of Clinical Physiology, Danderyds Hospital, S–18 288 Danderyd-Stockholm (Sweden)

Blaufox MD, Hollenberg NK, Raynaud C (eds): Radionuclides in Nephro-Urology.
Contrib Nephrol. Basel, Karger, 1990, vol 79, pp 21–23

Preliminary Results Comparing the Extraction Efficiencies of ^{131}I-OIH and ^{99m}Tc-MAG$_3$ in Rat Models of Ischemia, Renal Artery Stenosis, and Ciclosporin Toxicity[1]

Andrew Taylor, Jr., John Greene, Dennis Eshima, Dirck Dillehay[2]
Department of Radiology, Division of Nuclear Medicine,
Emory University School of Medicine, Atlanta, Ga., USA

During constant infusion plasma clearance studies, the clearance is measured by dividing the timed urine excretion of the tracer by plasma concentration. If the extraction efficiency is 100%, then the clearance is the renal plasma flow. Iodine-131 *o*-iodohippuran (^{131}I-OIH) and technetium-99m mercaptoacetyltriglycine (^{99m}Tc-MAG$_3$) clearances have been described as indices of renal plasma flow [1–5]. This assertion is true provided the extraction efficiency is high as reported for ^{131}I-OIH or at least remains constant; if the extraction fraction is constant, clearance is dependent upon and proportional to renal plasma flow. A recent report by Wenting et al. [6] indicated that the extraction fraction of OIH may fall in patients with renal artery stenosis receiving captopril. To the extent this is true, clinicians need to be aware that the measured OIH clearance, the 'effective renal plasma flow' may not be proportional to the true renal plasma flow. To determine the potential dissociation between ERPF and renal plasma flow for MAG$_3$ and OIH, we measured the renal extraction of ^{131}I-OIH, ^{99m}Tc-MAG$_3$ and a GFR reference agent ^{125}I-iothalamate (Ioth) in control rats and rats with ciclosporin toxicity, ischemia and acute renal artery stenosis.

Methods

The general methods we have utilized have been described previously [7, 8]. Three studies were conducted with separate controls for each group of experimental rats. Sprague-Dawley rats were used for the ischemic and renal artery stenosis (RAS) models and Fisher 344

[1] Supported by the National Institutes of Health, RO1 AM 33692.
[2] We wish to express our appreciation to Nan Harrison and Regina Lee for their secretarial assistance.

Table 1. Extraction efficiency of ^{99m}Tc-MAG_3, ^{131}I-OIH and ^{125}I-iothalomate as a percent of control in animal models of ciclosporin toxicity, ischemia and RAS

Animal model	Percent of control		
	MAG_3	OIH	Ioth
Ciclosporin toxicity	89	88	88
24 h postischemia	62	65	42
60% RAS	68	62	27

rats were used for the ciclosporin toxicity studies. The animals were prepared surgically as follows: a midline incision was made and the left renal artery was isolated; the core temperature was allowed to return to normal, 50 units of heparin were given intravenously through the femoral vein and 1 min later the left renal artery was occluded. The animals were closed and the core temperature maintained for the 30 min ischemic period. At the end of the ischemic period a right nephrectomy was performed. The control animals underwent an identical procedure; however, the left renal artery was not occluded. In the RAS model, a midline incision was made and the left renal artery isolated. Blood flow was determined using a square wave electromagnetic flowmeter and flow was then reduced by approximately 60% by partially occluding the renal artery with a silk ligature. The silk ligature was left in place and the animals were studied 24 h later following confirmation of approximately a 60% reduction in blood flow. Ciclosporin toxicity was induced by giving Fisher 344 rats 50 mg/kg of ciclosporin twice a day for 5 days. The ciclosporin was administered via a gastrostomy tube and the rats were studied on the sixth day.

Surgical procedures for the constant infusion clearance studies included a tracheostomy, cannulation of one jugular vein with two lines (one for constant infusion of the radiopharmaceutical agents and one for the saline infusion), cannulation of the carotid artery and catheterization of the bladder for urine collections. The animals received an intravenous infusion of ^{131}I-OIH, ^{99m}Tc-MAG_3 and ^{125}I-iothalamate to obtain steady-state blood levels. At the end of the infusion period a renal vein blood sample and a carotid artery blood sample were obtained. The blood samples were centrifuged at the end of the study for determination of the extraction efficiency. No correction was made for ^{131}I-OIH leakage out of the red cells.

The HPLC formulation of ^{99m}Tc-MAG_3 was prepared as previously described [7]. Briefly, the ^{99m}Tc complex was radiolabeled by dissolving 0.5–1.0 mg of the benzoate-protected ligand in 100 μl of a 1 *M* NaOH solution. One milliliter of ^{99m}Tc-pertechnetate in 0.9% saline was added to the benzoate-protected ligand solution followed by 1 mg (20 μl of a 50 mg/ml solution) of freshly prepared sodium dithionite. The mixture was heated at 82 °C for 5–10 min and the final preparation was purified by HPLC utilizing a C-18 ODS reverse phase column with a 4% ethanol/0.01 *M* sodium phosphate buffer at pH 7.0 as the mobile phase.

Results

The results of the extraction efficiency studies are listed in table 1 and show a significant decrease in extraction efficiency of all three agents in the ischemic and RAS models. The slight decrease in extraction fraction in the animals with ciclosporin toxicity was not statistically significant.

Discussion

The extraction efficiency of ^{99m}Tc-MAG$_3$ and ^{131}I-OIH decreased in animals with RAS and ischemia. The fall in extraction efficiency indicates that effective renal plasma flow as measured by ^{131}I-OIH and ^{99m}Tc-MAG$_3$ clearance may vary in its proportionality to renal plasma flow in these models. Importantly, however, the extraction efficiencies of ^{99m}Tc-MAG$_3$ and ^{131}I-OIH decreased comparably in all three models further supporting the use of ^{99m}Tc-MAG$_3$ as an ^{131}I-OIH replacement.

References

1 Tauxe WN, Maher FT, Taylor WM: Effective renal plasma flow: Estimation from theoretical volumes of distribution of intravenously injected ^{131}I-orthoiodohippurate. Mayo Clin Proc 1971;46:524–531.

2 Taylor A, Ziffer JA, Steves A, et al: Clinical comparision of ^{131}I-OIH and the kit formulation of ^{99m}Tc-mercaptoacetyltriglycine. Radiology 1989;170:721–725.

3 Jafri RA, Britton KE, Nimmon CC, et al: Technetium-99m MAG$_3$, a comparison with iodine-123 and iodine-131 orthoiodohippurate in patients with renal disorders. J Nucl Med 1988;29:147–158.

4 Russell CD, Thorstad B, Yester MV, et al: Comparison of technetium-99m MAG$_3$ with iodine-131 hippuran by a simultaneous dual channel technique. J Nucl Med 1988;29:1189–1193.

5 Bubeck B, Brandau W, Steinbacher M, et al: Technetium-99m labeled renal function agents. II. Clinical evaluation of Tc-99m MAG$_3$ (Tc-99 mercaptoacetylglycylglycylglycine). Nucl Med Biol 1988;15:109–118.

6 Wenting GL, Tan-Tjoing HL, Derky FHM, et al: Split renal function after captopril in unilateral renal artery stenosis. Hypertension 1984;6:I193–I197.

7 Eshima D, Taylor A, Fritzberg AR, et al: Animal evaluation of technetium-99m triamide mercaptide complexes as potential renal imaging agents. J Nucl Med 1987;28:1180–1186.

8 Taylor A, Eshima D: Effects of altered physiologic states on clearance and biodistribution of technetium-99m MAG$_3$, iodine-131 OIH, and iodine-125 iothalamate. J Nucl Med 1988;29:669-675.

Andrew Taylor, Jr., MD, Emory University Hospital,
Department of Radiology, Division of Nuclear Medicine, 1364 Clifton Road, NE,
Atlanta, GA 30350 (USA)

Blaufox MD, Hollenberg NK, Raynaud C (eds): Radionuclides in Nephro-Urology.
Contrib Nephrol. Basel, Karger, 1990, vol 79, pp 24–27

Preliminary Results Comparing OIH, ^{99m}Tc-MAG_3 and Iothalamate in a Rat Model of Renal Ischemia

Dennis Eshima, John Greene, Andrew Taylor, Jr.[1]

Department of Radiology, Division of Nuclear Medicine,
Emory University School of Medicine, Atlanta, Ga., USA

Technetium-99m mercaptoacetyltriglycine (^{99m}Tc-MAG_3) is a new renal tubular function agent which has shown promise as a replacement for ^{131}I *o*-iodohippurate (^{131}I-OIH) [1–4]. A simple kit formulation has been developed and is commercially available in Europe with a 1-hour shelf life postreconstitution. A more stable kit formulation has currently finished Phase III testing in the United States with a shelf life of 6 h [4, 5]. ^{99m}Tc-MAG_3 will probably replace ^{131}I-OIH for routine clinical studies including renal transplant evaluation. Since ischemic injury is a common problem in renal transplantation, we studied the effects of ischemic injury on the renal clearances of ^{131}I-OIH, ^{99m}Tc-MAG_3 and ^{125}I-iothalamate (Ioth) in an animal model.

Methods

The methods used in this study have been described previously in detail [6, 7]. Briefly, four groups of animals were studied, a sham ischemic single kidney control group and groups studied immediately and at 24 and 72 h after release of the clamp. The animals were prepared surgically as follows: a midline incision was made and the left renal artery was isolated; the core temperature was allowed to return to normal, then 50 units of heparin were given intravenously through the femoral vein and 1 min later the left renal artery was occluded. The animals were closed and the core temperature maintained for the 30-min ischemic period. At the end of the ischemic period a right nephrectomy was performed. The control animals underwent an identical procedure; however, the left renal artery was not occluded. The experimental animals were studied immediately and at 24 and 72 h after release of the clamp.

[1]The authors would like to acknowledge support from the National Institutes of Health R01 DK38842–93A1.

Table 1. ^{131}I-OIH, ^{99m}Tc-MAG_3 and ^{125}I-iothalamate clearances as a percent of the control value immediately and at 24 and 72 h postischemia

	Immediately	24 h	72 h
OIH	30.6	74.7	91.3
MAG_3	21.8	86.5	99.3
Ioth	20.8	56.6	111.3

Table 2. ^{99m}Tc-MAG_3/^{131}I-OIH and ^{125}I-iothalamate/^{131}I-OIH ratio of mean clearances of control and ischemic animals (% values)

	Control	Immediately	24 h	72 h
MAG_3/OIH	76	54	73	83
Ioth/OIH	29	19	22	35

Surgical procedures for the constant infusion clearance studies included a tracheostomy, cannulation of one jugular vein with two lines (one for constant infusion of the radiopharmaceutical agents and one for the saline infusion), cannulation of the carotid artery and catheterization of the bladder for urine collections. The animals were infused for 45 min to obtain steady-state levels followed by three 10-min urine collections with an arterial sample obtained during the midpoint of the urine collection period. The blood sample was centrifuged at the end of the study and a plasma sample was obtained for determination of the constant infusion clearance value.

The HPLC formulation of ^{99m}Tc-MAG_3 was prepared as previously described [7]. Briefly, the ^{99m}Tc complex was radiolabeled by dissolving 0.5–1.0 mg of the benzoate-protected ligand in 100 µl of a 1*M* NaOH solution. One milliliter of technetium-99m pertechnetate in 0.9% saline was added to the benzoate -protected ligand solution followed by 1 mg (20 µl of a 50 mg/ml solution) of freshly prepared sodium dithionite. The mixture was heated at 82 °C for 5–10 min and the final preparation was purified by HPLC utilizing a C-18 ODS reverse phase column with a 4% ethanol/0.01 *M* sodium phosphate buffer at pH 7.0 as the mobile phase.

Results

The renal clearances as a percent of control are listed in table 1. Compared to the control group there was a significant decrease in the renal clearance of all three agents immediately post release and 24 h after the ischemic period ($p < 0.05$); by 72 h the clearance values had essentially returned to original levels, however there was significant variability in the clearance data for individual animals within the 72-hour group. The range for ^{99m}Tc-MAG_3 clearances was 0.54–2.58 ml/min/100 g, 0.70–2.99 ml/min/100 g for ^{131}I-OIH and 0.16–1.34 ml/min/100 g for ^{125}I-iothalamate. A comparison of the ^{99m}Tc-MAG_3/^{131}I-OIH and Ioth/^{131}I-OIH clearance ratios are listed in table 2. The ^{99m}Tc-MAG_3/OIH and Ioth/OIH ratios were significantly less ($p < 0.05$) than control immediately after the ischemic period but the ratios returned to control values by 24 h. Ischemia did not significantly affect the plasma protein binding of the radiopharmaceuticals in any of the four groups of animals.

Discussion

^{99m}Tc-MAG_3 is a promising replacement for ^{131}I-OIH, however, it has demonstrated different pharmacokinetic parameters [1–5, 8, 9]. It is therefore important to compare the two agents in various well-defined disease models to determine if the differences are clinically significant. The ^{99m}Tc-MAG_3 clearances were more adversely affected than ^{131}I-OIH clearances in severe acute ischemic injury, possibly due to a lower affinity of ^{99m}Tc-MAG_3 for the tubular transport protein or due to the possibility that a higher percentage of ^{99m}Tc-MAG_3 is cleared by the proximal tubular cells. When a correction is made for the proportion of ^{131}I-OIH and ^{99m}Tc-MAG_3 cleared by the glomerulus, the clearance of ^{131}I-OIH by the tubular cells at 24 h is still greater than the clearance of ^{99m}Tc-MAG_3. This study shows that although there may be minor differences between the two agents in acute ischemia, overall ^{99m}Tc-MAG_3 performs similarly to ^{131}I-OIH in ischemic injury.

References

1 Taylor A, Eshima D, Fritzberg AR, et al: Comparison of iodine-131 OIH and technetium-99m MAG_3 renal imaging in volunteers. J Nucl Med 1986;27:795–803.

2 Taylor A, Eshima D, Christian PE, et al: Evaluation of Tc-99m mercaptoacetyltriglycine in patients with impaired renal function. Radiology 1987;162:365–370.

3 Taylor A, Eshima D, Christian PE, et al: Technetium-99m MAG_3 kit formulation: Preliminary results in normal volunteers and patients with renal failure. J Nucl Med 1988;29:616–622.

4 Russell CD, Thorstad B, Yester MV, et al: Comparision of technetium-99m MAG_3 with iodine-131 hippuran by a simultaneous dual channel technique. J Nucl Med 1988;29:1189–1193.

5 Taylor A, Ziffer JA, Steves A, et al: Clinical comparison of I-131 orthoiodohippurate and the kit formulation of Tc-99m mercaptoacetyltriglycine. Radiology 1989;170:721–725.

6 Eshima D, Taylor A, Fritzberg AR, et al: Animal evaluation of technetium-99m triamide mercaptide complexes as potential renal imaging agents. J Nucl Med 1987;28:1180–1186.

7 Taylor A, Eshima D: Effects of altered physiologic states on clearance and biodistribution of technetium-99m MAG_3, iodine-131 OIH, and iodine-125 iothalamate. J Nucl Med 1988;29:669–675.
8 Taylor A, Eshima D, Alazraki N: $^{99m}Tc-MAG_3$, a new renal imaging agent: Preliminary results in patients. Eur J Nucl Med 1987;12:510–514.
9 Jafri RA, Britton KE, Nimmon CC, et al: Technetium-99m MAG_3, a comparison with iodine-123 and iodine-131 ortho-iodohippurate, in patients with renal disorders. J Nucl Med 1988;29:147–158.

Dennis Eshima, PhD, University of New Mexico, College of Pharmacy (Radiopharmacy), Albuquerque, NM 87131 (USA)

Blaufox MD, Hollenberg NK, Raynaud C (eds): Radionuclides in Nephro-Urology.
Contrib Nephrol. Basel, Karger, 1990, vol 79, pp 28–31

$^{99m}Tc-MAG_3$: A Routine Renal Radiopharmaceutical

K.E. Britton, S. Miceva, A.M. Al-Nahhas, R.A. Jafri, J. Bomanji, K. Solanki, M.J. Carroll, C.C. Nimmon

St. Bartholomew's Hospital, London, UK

^{99m}Tc mercaptoacetyltriglycine (MAG_3) is a new N3-S radiopharmaceutical developed by Frizberg et al. [1] that is tubularly secreted. The aim of this study was to test $^{99m}Tc-MAG_3$, supplied by Mallinckrodt Diagnostica Holland BV, in routine use as a replacement for previous radiopharmaceuticals for renal dynamic studies. ^{131}I orthoiodohippurate (OIH), ^{123}I-OIH, and ^{99m}Tc-DTPA. Our previous work [2] showed that there was a direct proportionality between the clearance of $^{99m}Tc-MAG_3$ and ^{131}I-OIH such that $OIH = 1.5\ MAG_3 + 40$ ml/min (SEE 8%) [3]. The lower clearance was due to the smaller volume of distribution of $^{99m}Tc-MAG_3$ by single [2] or biexponential analysis [4] being 0.65 that of ^{131}I-OIH, but a similar plasma half-life, 1.09 that of ^{131}I-OIH [2]. Protein binding was 78% for $^{99m}Tc-MAG_3$ as compared to 70% for ^{131}I-OIH [5]. Images obtained with $^{99m}Tc-MAG_3$ were as good as those with ^{123}I-OIH (each 2.5 mCi, 100 MBq injected) and better than those with ^{99m}Tc-DTPA (10 mCi, 400 MBq injected) particularly when renal function was poor and in renal transplants [2, 6]. It was also shown that the relative renal functions measured with $^{99m}Tc-MAG_3$ were highly correlated with those of ^{123}I-OIH, r 0.97, and with those of ^{99m}Tc-DTPA, r 0.94 (both $p < 0.001$). Frusemide responses with all agents were similar. Renal transit times were obtained by deconvolution analysis [7]. For obstructive nephropathy a value of the parenchymal transit time index (PTTI) over 156 s in its context of outflow disorder [8] and for renovascular disorder a value of the mean parenchymal transit time (MPTT) of over 240 s in the context of hypertension are abnormal [6]. Regression analysis of PTTI for $^{99m}Tc-MAG_3$ gave with ^{131}I-OIH, r 0.81 and with ^{99m}Tc-DTPA, r 0.87. Regression analysis of the whole kidney transit time index (WKTTI) [4] for $^{99m}Tc-MAG_3$ gave with ^{131}I-OIH, r 0.92 and with ^{99m}Tc-DTPA, r 0.97. Regression analysis of MPTT for $^{99m}Tc-MAG_3$ gave with ^{123}I-OIH, r 0.79 and with ^{99m}Tc-DTPA, r 0.78.

Method of Preparation

MAG_3 was supplied as a powder in sealed glass vials. Five millicuries (185 MBq) of ^{99m}Tc-04 was eluted from a Mallinckrodt technetium generator (code UTK) and volume dilution to the appropriate patient dose (100 MBq) was done with physiological saline. The vial was then placed in a lead-shielded boiling water bath for 10 min to remove the protective benzoyl group, then cooled under running tap water. The $^{99m}Tc-MAG_3$ prepared in this way must be used within 60 min to maintain 95% radiopharmaceutical purity, since there is a build up of lipophilic impurities which are taken up slowly by the liver to the extent of up to 4% of the injected dose. Solanki et al. [9] have applied the Arrhenius equation to the rate of reaction related to these impurities. They demonstrated that subsequent to the boiling step, freezing up to five aliquots of the preparation in syringes capped with blind hubs led to the maintenance of over 95% purity for over 8 h after preparation. The 'cold MAG_3' technique reduced the rate of build up of the impurities almost 100-fold from 0.4%/min (manufacturer's technique) to 0.006%/min. The syringe is rethawed before use under a table lamp when the patient arrives. Since this approach has been used routinely, liver uptake has virtually disappeared. A comparison of normal parenchymal transit times for the right and left kidneys showed no significant difference.

Patient Studies

Over 600 patients have been studied using $^{99m}Tc-MAG_3$ as the radiopharmaceutical for routine renal dynamic studies with a distribution of requests as follows: hypertension 41%; outflow disorder 33%; renal transplant 19%; miscellaneous 7%. No clinical side effects or problems have been noted. Since the introduction of the 'cold MAG_3' technique, liver uptake has been hardly evident. In oliguric patients with poor $^{99m}Tc-MAG_3$ uptake, no increase in any liver uptake has been observed. The qualtiy of results has been better than that previously seen with ^{99m}Tc-DTPA, particularly when renal function in one or both kidneys was impaired (fig. 1).

Dividing the preparation from one vial into aliquots, up to five patient doses per vial are obtained so that the cost per patient is not much greater than that for ^{99m}Tc-DTPA. However, this would apply only to a department with a high renal workload.

$^{99m}Tc-MAG_3$ is excellent for the evaluation of obstructive nephropathy using PTTI and WKTTI and the percentage outflow efficiency which relates a frusemide response to the level of renal function works well [10]. $^{99m}Tc-MAG_3$ has been used to evaluate renovascular disorder, using MPTT alone and with captopril. In essential hypertension, captopril causes no significant change of MPTT, but a slight increase occurs with large or small vessel disease causing renovascular disorder. Intrarenal flow distribution is also measureable. Better definition of the kidney is seen in renal trasplantation and the good statistical data makes it easier to obtain a reliable perfusion index.

In conclusion, $^{99m}Tc-MAG_3$ combines the availability, high count rate qualities and convenience of the technetium label with the physiological advantages of a hippuran-like compound and is excellent for routine renal dynamic studies in a department with an active nephrourological commitment.

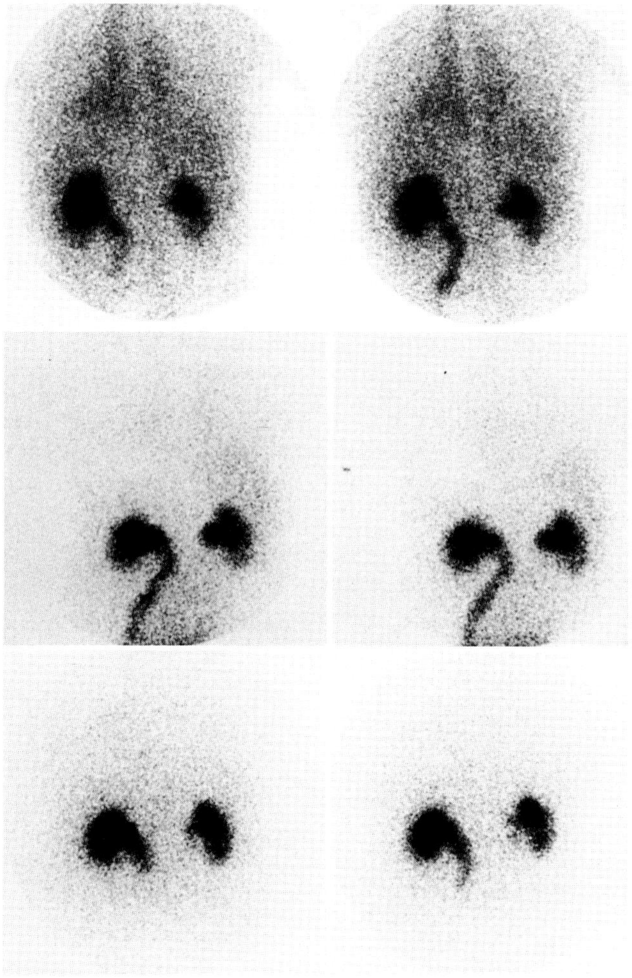

Fig. 1. Bilateral obstructive nephropathy, creatinine clearance 15 ml/min. Posterior 15- and 20-min images. *a* ^{99m}Tc-DPTA (10 mCi, 400 MBq). *b* ^{99m}Tc-MAG_3 (2.5 mCi, 100 MBq). *c* ^{123}I-OIH (2.5 mCi, 100 MBq). The high tissue blood and liver background with ^{99m}Tc-DTPA is evident. The slight liver background with ^{99m}Tc-MAG_3 has been reduced further by the 'cold MAG_3' technique (see text).

References

1 Fritzberg AR, Kasina S, Eshima DL, et al: Synthesis and biological evaluation of technetium-99m MAG_3 as a hippuran replacement. J Nucl Med 1986;27:111–116.

2 Jafri RA, Britton KE, Nimmon CC, et al: ^{99m}Tc-MAG_3, a comparison with I-123 and I-131 orthoiodohippurate in patients with renal disorders. J Nucl Med 1988;29:147–158.

3 Britton KE, Jafri RA, Nimmon CC: Comparison of the clearance of technetium-99m-MAG_3 and iodine-131-OIH. J Nucl Med 1988;29:1878–1879.

4 Nimmon CC, Britton KE, Al-Nahhas A, et al: ^{99m}Tc-MAG_3 (mercaptoacetyltriglycine): a renal pharaceutical for routine use; in dynamic functional studies in Nuclear Medicine in Developing Countries. Vienna, International Atomic Energy Agency, 1989.

5 Britton KE, Brown NJG: Clinical Renography. London, Lloyd Luke Ltd, 1971.

6 Al-Nahhas AA, Jafri RA, Britton KE, et al: Clinical experience with ^{99m}Tc-MAG_3, mercaptoacetyltriglycine, and a comparison with ^{99m}Tc-DTPA. Eur J Nucl Med 1988;14:453–462.

6 Al-Nahhas AA, Jafri RA, Britton KE, et al: Clinical experience with ^{99m}Tc-MAG_3, mercaptoacetyltriglycine, and a comparison with ^{99m}Tc-DTPA. Eur J Nucl Med 1988;14:453–462.

7 Britton KE, Maisey MN: Renal radionuclide studies; in Maisey MN, Britton KE, Gilday DL (eds): Clinical Nuclear Medicine. London, Chapman & Hall, 1983, pp 93–120.

8 Britton KE, Nawaz MK, Whitfield HN, et al: Obstructive nephropathy: comparison between parenchymal transit index and frusemide diuresis. Br J Urol 1987;59:127–132.

9 Solanki KK, Al-Nahhas AA, Britton KE: 'Cold' ^{99m}Tc-MAG_3; in Schmidt HAE, Buraggi GL (eds): Nuclear Medicine. Proc Eur Nucl Med Congr, Milan 1988. Stuttgart, Schattauer, 1989, pp 443–446.

10 Nimmon CC, Britton KE, Bomanji, J. et al: Quantitation of Frusemide response, with a comparison with parenchymal transit time analysis in the ^{99m}Tc-DTPA renal study; in Schmidt HAE, Csernay L (eds): Nuklearmedizin: New Trends and Possibilities in Nuclear Medicine. Proc Eur Nucl Med Congr, Budapest 1987. Stuttgart, Schattauer, 1988, pp 472–475.

K.E. Britton, MD, Department of Nuclear Medicine, St. Bartholomew's Hospital, West Smithfield, London EC19 7BE (UK)

Blaufox MD, Hollenberg NK, Raynaud C (eds): Radionuclides in Nephro-Urology.
Contrib Nephrol. Basel, Karger, 1990, vol 79, pp 32–35

A Comparative Study of Renal Scintigraphy and Clearance with ^{99m}Tc-MAG$_3$ and ^{123}I-Hippurate in Patients with Renal Disorders

Roland Müller-Suur [a], *Ingeborg Bois-Svensson* [b], *Laszlo Mesko* [b]

[a] Karolinska Institute, Department of Clinical Physiology, Danderyds Hospital;
[b] Department of Hospital Physics, Danderyds Hospital, Stockholm, Sweden

Recently a new radiopharmaceutical for renal dynamic scintigraphy, ^{99m}Tc-mercaptoacetyltriglycine (MAG$_3$) has been introduced [1] which combines the advantage of high renal extraction with a desirable energy emission for gamma camera imaging. In rat experiments [2] some excretion characteristics of MAG$_3$ in comparison with hippurate have been outlined and first clinical trials have been reported [3–6]. The present clinical trial was performed to compare MAG$_3$ with ^{123}I-hippurate (^{123}I-OIH) since the physical properties of ^{99m}Tc and ^{123}I are similar. We also wanted to study whether the observation in rats of a significant extrarenal excretion to the bile [2] is present in patients.

Methods

Seventeen patients were studied. All were referred for evaluation of different nephrourological disorders and first investigated with our routine ^{123}I-hippuran gamma camera renography and participated in an additional renography with ^{99m}Tc-MAG$_3$ 2–8 days later. For the first study, 1 mCi (37 MBq) ^{123}I-hippurate (Radio Isotopenservice, Würenlingen, Switzerland) was used, and for the second study 2 mCi (70 MBq) ^{99m}Tc-MAG$_3$ (kit prepared by Mallinckrodt, Petten, The Netherlands). The radiochemical purity was according to the manufacturer $>95\%$. For ^{123}I-hippurate, the plasma clearance was calculated according to Tauxe and Dubovsky [7], i.e. a 44-min one-sample 'ERPF' method. For ^{99m}Tc-MAG$_3$ clearance, six venous plasma samples at 5, 10, 20, 44, 60 and 120 min postinjection were taken from the forearm opposite to the injection arm. MAG$_3$ clearance was calculated from the injected amount divided by the area under the curve of plasma activity versus time. For calculation of urine excretion the patients were asked to void 60 min postinjection and urine analyzed. The excretion was then expressed as percent of the injected amount. For estimation of blood cell content in percent of whole blood activity, blood was counted using the 44-min samples and corrected for plasma activity and hematocrit.

Gamma camera data were collected in 2.5 s frame mode by a computer system. Dynamic pictures were collected at 20 min and additional dorsal pictures were, if possible and convenient for the patient, collected at 60–62 and 120–122 min postinjection. Conventional renograms were created, corrected for depth of the kidneys (ultrasound) and the individual semilunar backgrounds from which the relative renal function, i.e. 1–3 min uptake, was calculated. The liver and spleen uptake was determined as the ratio of activity per pixel of liver or spleen region to the activity per pixel of the background region (aorta). Ureteral peristalsis was displayed on a time space matrix as described by Müller-Schauenburg et al. [8] using a special software for the gamma 11 computer.

Results and Discussion

(1) The clearance of ^{123}I-OIH ranged from 10 to 654, whereas that of MAG_3 from 15 to 328 ml/min 1.73 m^2 which was significantly lower ($p < 0.001$), $59 \pm 7\%$ that of ^{123}I-OIH. The correlation was high: $y = 26.13 \pm 0.44x$, $r = 0.92$, $p < 0.001$. (2) The rate of urinary excretion at 60 min was not significantly different between MAG_3 and ^{123}I-OIH. (3) The 44 min distribution of MAG_3 was significantly lower, range 14–49 liters, than that of ^{123}I-OIH, range 17–136 liters, but correlated well, $r = 0.82$, $p < 0.001$. (4) The activity of MAG_3 in blood cells was $7.4 \pm 1\%$ of the whole blood activity as compared to $26.9 \pm 3.5\%$ for ^{123}I-OIH ($p < 0.01$), whereas the plasma protein binding of MAG_3 was 90 ± 2 and that of ^{123}I-OIH $74 \pm 2\%$ ($p < 0.05$) as measured by a centrifugation filtration technique (Centrifree; Amicon, Mass., USA). This argues for restricted glomerular filtration as demonstrated in rat glomeruli [9] also in humans. (5) The gamma camera images looked quite similar using MAG_3 or ^{123}I-OIH. Figure 1 shows an example. (6) Ureteral peristalsis, if visible in the baseline study with ^{123}I-OIH, could also be displayed using MAG_3. Figure 1 shows peristaltic waves more clearly using MAG_3. (7) Liver uptake of MAG_3 increased with time and was significantly higher at 18–20 min ($p < 0.001$) than that of ^{123}I-OIH, ranging 1.00–2.40 times that of the aorta background (range for ^{123}I-OIH was 0.77–1.30). It was not related to kidney function. The background to kidney ratio at 2–4 min was the same for both tracers. (8) From the renograms the calculated relative individual kidney functions were the same for MAG_3 or ^{123}I-OIH, also the time to peak activity was not different. But the elimination of MAG_3 from the kidneys was slower measured as elimination ratio (activity 10 min after peak activity) and also as time to 50% of peak activity. This was evidently not explained by different urine flow rates. Slower MAG_3 elimination is evident also in the example given in figure 1.

Most of our findings are in accordance with earlier reports [2–4, 6]. One study [5] using HPLC-purified MAG_3 did not observe liver uptake,

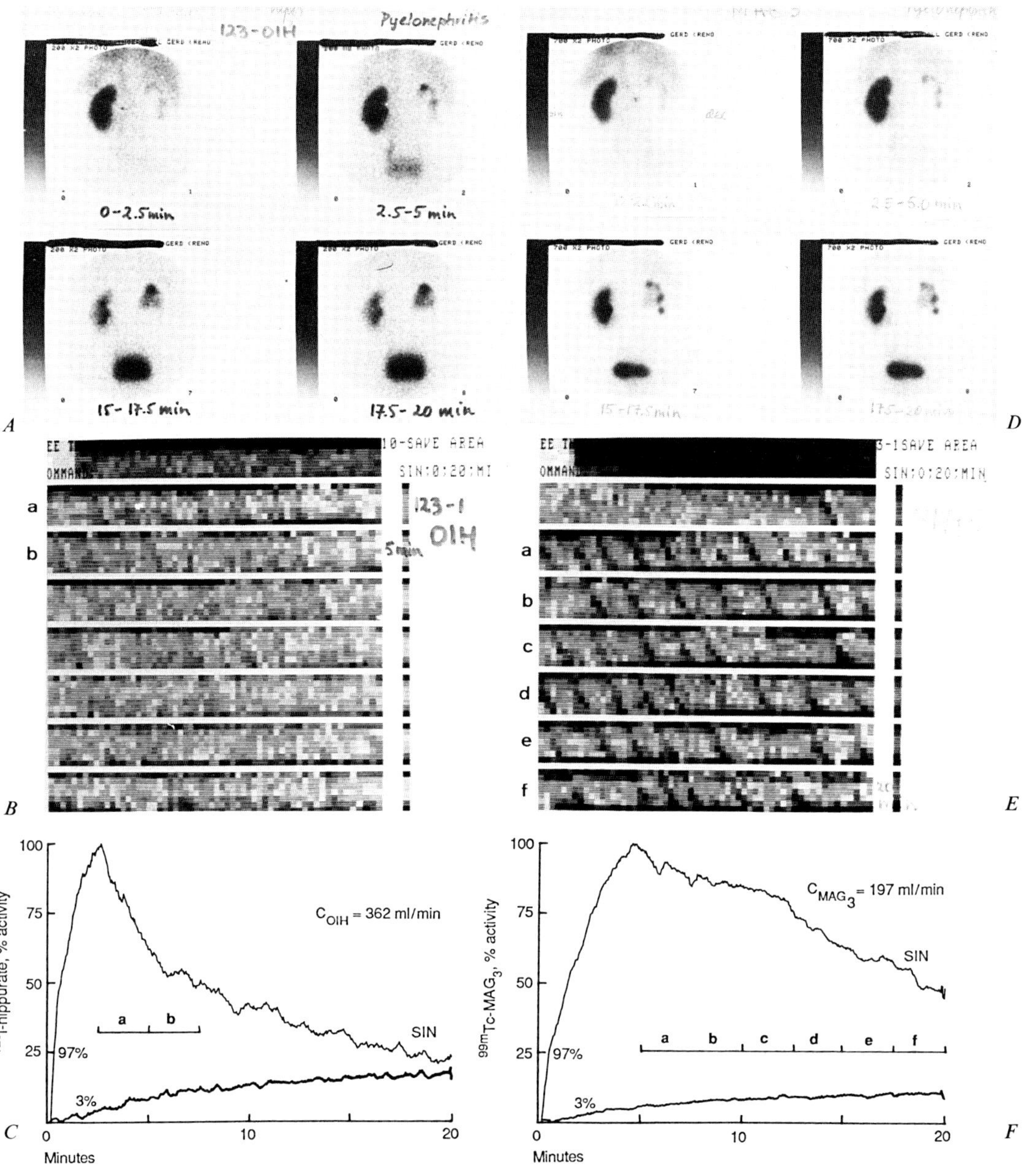

Fig. 1. Images *(A,D)*, time-space matrix *(B,E)* and renograms *(C,F)* of a patient with earlier pyelonephritis referred for evaluation of right kidney separate function, which is 3% in both the ^{123}I-hippurate study *(A–C)* and the MAG_3 study *(D–F)*. Activity lines in the time-space matrix indicating peristaltic contractions of the left ureter are seen in both studies, but more clearly using MAG_3 (see rows a–f in *E* corresponding to 5–20 min postinjection, *F*) than using ^{123}I-hippurate (see rows a and b in *B*, i.e. 2.5–7.5 min postinjection, *C*).

whereas it was seen by others [2–4, 6] and also in the present study. Since it is rather low and significant only in late images it does not jeopardize reliable calculation of right kidney function. However, the exact amount of such extrarenal clearance is unclear and variable. Secretion occurs with both tracers in the kidneys although of a lower magnitude for MAG_3 [9] and there is a more restricted filtration of MAG_3 than of hippurate in the glomerulus [9] which results in lower renal extraction [2] and clearance of MAG_3 than hippurate [2–6]. This together with estimation errors for MAG_3 clearance argues against its use in measuring renal plasma flow.

References

1 Fritzberg AR, Kasima S, Eshima D, et al: Synthesis and biologic evaluation of technetium-99m-MAG_3 as a hippuran replacement. J Nucl Med 1986;27:111–116.

2 Müller-Suur R, Müller-Suur C: Renal and extrarenal handling of a new imaging compound (^{99m}Tc-MAG_3) in the rat. Eur J Nucl Med 1986; 27:111:442.

3 Jafri AR, Britton KE, Nimmon CE, et al: Technetium-99m-MAG_3, a comparison with iodine-123 and diodine-131-orthoidohippurate in patients with renal disorders. J Nucl Med 1988;29:147–158.

4 Taylor A, Ziffer JA, Stevens A, et al: Clinical comparison of ^{131}I-orthoiodohippurate and the kit formulation of ^{99m}Tc-mercaptoacetyltriglycine. Radiology 1989;170:721–725.

5 Brandau W, Bubeck B, Berger J, et al: Excretion characteristics of ^{99m}Tc-MAG_3 in patients; in Schmidt HEA, Buraggi GL (eds): Nuclear Medicine. Stuttgart, Schattauer, 1989, pp 409–412.

6 Martin WG, Wolf IH, Kempken K, et al: ^{99m}Tc-MAG_3 versus ^{123}I-OIH: Comparison of quantitative parameters in renal function; in Schmidt HEA, Buraggi GL (eds): Nuclear Medicine, Stuttgart, Schattauer, 1989, pp 413–416.

7 Tauxe WN, Dubovsky EV, Kidd TE: Comparison of measurement of effective renal plasma flow by single plasma sample and plasma disappearance slope/volume methods. Eur J Nucl Med 1985;9:443–445.

8 Müller-Schauenburg W, Hofmann U, Feine U, et al: Criteria for ureteral obstruction by functional imaging of the upper urinary tract. Contrib Nephrol 1987;56:225–231.

9 Müller-Suur C, Müller-Suur R: Handling of ^{99m}Tc-MAG_3 in the kidney; in Blaufox DM, Hollenberg NK, Raynaud C: Radionuclides in Nephro-Urology. Contrib Nephrol. Basel, Karger, 1990, vol 79, pp 17–20.

Roland Müller-Suur, MD, Karolinska Institute, Department of Clinical Physiology, Danderyds Hospital, S–18 288 Danderyd-Stockholm (Sweden)

Blaufox MD, Hollenberg NK, Raynaud C (eds): Radionuclides in Nephro-Urology.
Contrib Nephrol. Basel, Karger, 1990, vol 79, pp 36–40

Renal Imaging of Thallium-201 during Cardiac Evaluation

Naomi P. Alazraki, Jack A. Ziffer, William Fajman, James Galt, Raghu Halkar, Linda Hanna

Emory University School of Medicine and Veterans Administration Medical Center, Atlanta, Ga., USA

Thallium-201 myocardial perfusion imaging studies are widely performed combined with treadmill electrocardiographic stress testing for suspected coronary artery disease. Patients with coronary artery disease have an increased incidence of renal and peripheral vascular disease, as well as hypertension. Thallium, following intravenous administration, distributes to all parts of the body in relation to the regional blood flow. The heart receives approximately 3–5% of the total cardiac output and approximately 3–5% of the injected thallium chloride dose. The kidneys are the major route of excretion of thallium from the body, and in fact the critical organ, receiving the highest radiation dose from thallium-201 [1].

The purpose of this study was to assess the value of a routine image of the kidneys to detect occult renovascular disease following stress thallium imaging in patients being evaluated for coronary artery disease.

Methods

The study population consisted of 123 consecutive patients referred to the nuclear medicine departments at two institutions in Atlanta: The Grady Memorial, a county hospital (100 patients), and the Veterans Administration Medical Center (23 patients), for evaluation of coronary artery disease by thallium-201 treadmill stress of dipyridamole imaging. There were 68 women and 55 men studied at the two institutions.

Twenty patients had intravenous dipyridamole (0.726 mg/kg) and 103 were stressed on a treadmill under cardiology supervision. At peak stress, or immediately following a 5-min dipyridamole infusion, 3.5 mCi of thallium-201 chloride was injected intravenously, followed immediately and at 180 min postinjection by SPECT imaging which took 22 min per acquisition. Following SPECT acquisition of cardiac images, 500,000 counts were acquired from a posterior abdominal projection using planar scintillation camera imaging. The large-field camera had a low-energy all-purpose parallel-hole collimator and its pulse height analyzers were set using a 20% window centered at 72 keV.

Image Analysis. Relative activity in the two kidneys was assessed by visual interpretation and by background-corrected computer analysis. A range of 40–60% uptake in either kidney was considered within normal limits. Asymmetric uptake, defined as less than 40% uptake in either kidney, was considered abnormal.

Patient Data Analysis. Patients' clinical and radiographic histories were reviewed retrospectively. The thallium renal uptake findings were correlated with recent radiographic studies including renal angiograms, renal ultrasound, renal computed tomography and intravenous pyelography.

Results

Renal thallium uptake studies were normal in 93 cases. Of those, 35 had other renal imaging studies (ultrasound, computer tomography, or intravenous pyelography). Seven abnormal results were identified, including cysts, scarring, infarction, hydronephrosis, and asymmetric renal size. Three of 93 normal renal thallium subjects had angiography of the kidneys. One renal tumor and two normal renal angiograms were identified. There were 30 abnormal thallium renal studies. Among these, 4 patients had renal angiography. Three had renal vascular disease (fig. 1a, b) and one had ureteral obstruction. Fourteen patients had other renal imaging studies (ultrasound, intravenous pyelography, computed tomography). Twelve of the 14 were abnormal and showed cysts, scarring, infarction, hydronephrosis, infiltrative processes, nephrectomy, or atrophy. Among the 123 patients studied, 75 had hypertension. Twenty-seven of the patients with hypertension (36%) had abnormal thallium renal studies. Forty-eight of the patients with hypertension (64%) had normal thallium renal studies. Eighteen of 30 abnormal thallium renal studies had radiographic correlation, which showed an abnormality in 16 (89%) of the 18. Thirty-eight of the 93 normal thallium renal studies had radiographic correlation. Eight (21%) of those 38 had an abnormality demonstrated.

Discussion

The results of this study indicated a large disparity in renal abnormalities (parenchymal or renal vascular) identified by other imaging techniques in patients who had abnormal versus normal thallium renal uptake (89% vs. 21%). Sensitivity and specificity of abnormal thallium renal uptake cannot be accurately determined from this study because it is retrospective and there was incomplete evaluation of patients for sensitivity, specificity determinations.

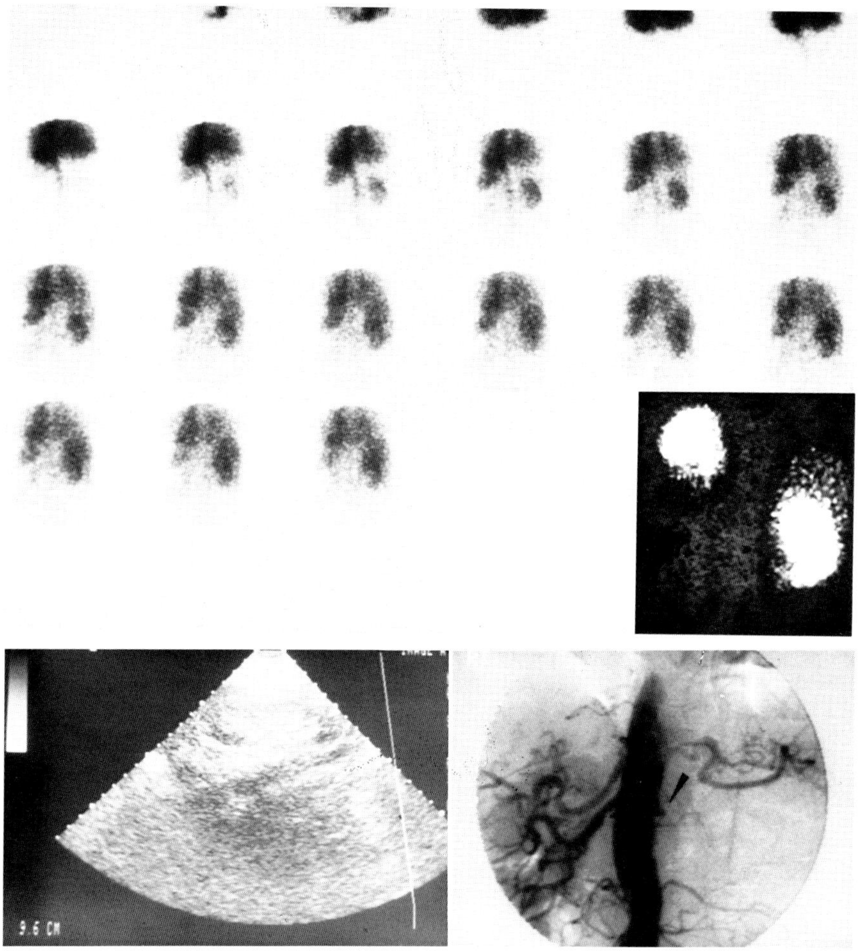

a

b

Fig. 1. *a* ^{99m}Tc-DTPA sequential images at 2 s/frame following intravenous injection and 1–2 min image (lower right) show no perfusion or uptake in the left kidney. Large insert photo at bottom right shows thallium in the right kidney, none in the left kidney, and thallium in the myocardium. *b* Ultrasound shows presence of a small kidney and radiographic aortogram shows only a nubbin of a left renal artery (arrow) which is totally occluded.

Clorious and Schmidlin [2] demonstrated that stress renography using ^{99m}Tc-DTPA and/or ^{131}I-hippuran showed more renal abnormalities than conventional renography performed at rest. In the current study, renal thallium images were performed at approximately 25 min following completion of treadmill exercise or dipyridamole injection. Alterations in cortical renal blood flow have been shown with exercise in hypertensive subjects and a correlation with hypertension and abnormal renal thallium uptake could theoretically be augmented by the poststress imaging procedure.

Radiologists have made a practice of routinely imaging the kidneys following contrast angiography of other organs or vessels. Particularly because of the high association between renal vascular disease, hypertension and coronary artery disease, it would seem reasonable to image the thallium renal distribution following thallium myocardial perfusion imaging in patients being evaluated for coronary artery disease. The results of this study, performed in a population with a high incidence of hypertension, indicates high yield of abnormal renal findings, attributable to both parenchymal and renal vascular etiologies. Since thallium has been shown to distribute in proportion to cardiac output to the kidneys [3], indeed the uptake distributions correlated with renal blood flow as well as parenchymal integrity since uptake of the thallium depends upon viability of cortical and medullary cells. In fact, thallium has a net extraction of 90% during its transrenal passage, with slightly lower extraction fractions measured in higher blood flow zones of the kidney [3].

Raynaud et al. [4] studied thallium distribution in rabbit kidneys and reported a 4:1 ratio of thallium in the medulla relative to the cortex. Their studies were performed using thallium-EDTA rather than thallium chloride which is the chemical form widely used for myocardial imaging. More importantly, Raynaud et al. [4] showed that the thallium distribution within the kidney changes with time, both in terms of global uptake and relative cortex to medulla uptake. We know from many renal studies of relative uptake of ^{99m}Tc-DTPA and iodohippuran that the most reliable time to record relative uptake as an indicator of relative blood flow and split renal function is at 1–3 min following intravenous injection [5–7]. Unfortunately, we cannot obtain the thallium renal images until 22–25 min after thallium injection, because of the need for immediate cardiac imaging. Thus, the real significance of the relative renal thallium counts obtained at 25 min or 4 h after thallium injection is not known.

Abnormal thallium uptake in the kidneys may be seen in renal vascular and/or renal parenchymal disease. A routine image of the kidneys following thallium myocardial perfusion imaging in patients referred because of possible coronary artery disease appears to be beneficial to detect occult renal vascular or parenchymal disease.

References

1 Strauss HW, Harrison K, Pitt B: Thallium-201: Non-invasive determination of the regional distribution of cardiac output. J Nucl Med 1977;18:1167–1170.

2 Clorius JH, Schmidlin P: The exercise renogram. A new approach documents renal involvement in systemic hypertension. J Nucl Med 1983;24:104–109.

3 Abildgaard U, Amtorp O, Gyring J, et al: Intrarenal blood flow distribution in dog kidney determined by ^{99m}Tc microaggregates and ^{201}Tl. Am J Physiol (Heart Circ Physiol 24) 1988;255:H1535–H1541.

4 Raynaud C, Ricard S, Comer D: ^{199}Tl uptake on the medulla of the kidney in man. Proc 3rd Int Symp on Radionuclides in Nephrology. Stuttgart, Thieme, 1975.

5 Gates GF: Glomerular filtration rate: estimation from fraction renal accumulation of ^{99m}Tc-DTPA (stannous). Am J Roentgenol 1982;138:565–570.

6 McAfee JG, Thomas FD, Subramanian G, et al: Detection of diffuse glomerular lesions in rats. I. Comparison of conventional radioactive agents. J Nucl Med 1986;27:502–512.

7 McAfee JG, Kopecky RT, Thomas FD, et al: Comparison of different radioactive agents for the detection of renovascular hypertension with captopril in a rat model. J Nucl Med 1988;29:509–515.

Naomi P. Alazraki, MD, Emory University School of Medicine and Veterans Administration Medical Center, Atlanta, GA 30322 (USA)

Blaufox MD, Hollenberg NK, Raynaud C (eds): Radionuclides in Nephro-Urology.
Contrib Nephrol. Basel, Karger, 1990, vol 79, pp 41–44

The Permeability of the Human Bladder to Water Assessed Using Tritiated Water

A.J.W. Hilson, C.A. Lewis, S.J. Harland
St. Peter's Hospital and Institute of Urology, London, UK

It is generally assumed that urine retrieved from the bladder is essentially identical to that excreted by the kidney, and this assumption is so basic that it is not even mentioned, let alone considered. However, Levinsky and Berliner [1] showed in 1959 that the flux of water, urea, and creatinine across the ureter and bladder of the dog was certainly not negligible, and Fellows and Marshall [2] showed that the human bladder, while poorly permeable to sodium, was very permeable to water (confirming work in other mammals). We have re-assessed this work in the context of possible changes in patients with bladder tumours.

Methods

We used the method of Fellows and Marshall [2]. The subjects were patients with differentiated bladder tumours who were being catheterized for intravesical chemotherapy. One normal volunteer also was studied on three occasions. After placement of a bladder catheter, the bladder was emptied. Between 130 and 200 ml of a sterile solution containing between 1.4 and 4.5 MBq of ^3H_2O was then infused into the bladder. It was left for about 40 min, during which time blood samples were taken, and then the bladder was emptied. The bladder was then filled with saline to assess the bladder capacity. A 'spike' of approximately 1.5 MBq of the same preparation of ^3H_2O was then injected intravenously, and blood samples obtained to estimate the volume of distribution, and hence the actual activity of ^3H_2O which was present in the blood during the instillation time. The water was extracted from the samples by vacuum distillation, and tritium activity estimated by liquid scintillation counting.

The study was approved by the Institute's Ethical Committee and by the Administration of Radiation Substances Advisory Committee (ARSAC).

Table 1. Absorption of ^3H_2O from the bladder in 9 subjects

Subject	Instilled		Absorbed		Time min	Bladder capacity, ml
	volume ml	MBq	MBq	%		
H.M.	198	1.44	0.122	8.5	35	455
H.K.	198	3.26	0.585	17.9	32	220
R.R.	148	3.50	0.406	11.6	35	360
A.O'M.	149	3.77	0.631	16.7	41.5	315
S.M.	200	4.21	0.387	9.2	40	700
F.B.	145	2.76	0.516	18.7	40	230
G.C.	130	3.40	0.650	19.1	42.5	260
I.R.	198	3.35	0.219	15.3	30	600
S.H.	198	2.21	0.526	23.8	42	690

Table 2. Absorption of ^3H_2O from the bladder of a normal volunteer at three different volumes: the bladder wall area is calculated assuming the bladder to be spherical; the units of transfer are $MBq \cdot ml \cdot cpm^{-1} \cdot min^{-1} \cdot 10^8$ (see text)

Volume, ml	Area, cm^2	Uptake, MBq	Time, min	Transfer
124	120	0.858	41.5	4.995
223	178	0.526	42	5.583
412	268	0.455	31	7.942

Results

The absorption from the bladder in the patients and the normal volunteer (S.H.) is shown in table 1. Table 2 shows the rate of transfer at different volumes in the normal volunteer. The units of transfer are $MBq \cdot ml \cdot cpm^{-1} \cdot min^{-1} \cdot 10^8$ to correct for varying activities and volumes instilled into the bladder, and the different times for which the fluid was left in the bladder.

Discussion

The degrees of transfer we have shown here are very similar to those of Fellows and Marshall [2] (who quote a figure of approximately 20% of the instilled activity per hour). They showed that the presence of well-differentiated tumours or previous radiotherapy did not significantly change the permeability. We have not calculated permeability for our subjects, in particular because it is necessary to assume the shape of the bladder. However, the highest transfer was seen in our normal volunteer.

Levinsky and Berliner [1] showed that, in the dog, movement of water and solutes occurred, and was in the direction of concentration gradients. They also showed that it was not affected by changes in antidiuretic hormone activity, anaesthesia, or surgical manipulation. Our data on a single volunteer at different volumes shows that the rate of transfer increases as the bladder volume, and presumably surface area, increases. This is certainly compatible with a passive diffusion process. Fellows' data, together with other work in our department, shows that the normal human bladder shows very poor sodium transport, so it is unlikely that the water is being co-transported with sodium.

We have only demonstrated a unidirectional flux of ^3H_2O. Since the volume recovered from the bladder was always greater than that instilled (no measures were adopted to suppress the subjects' urine flow), it is very unlikely that this is not a bidirectional flux. This also implies that this is a passive flux, and makes it even more likely that the caution of Levinsky and Berliner [1] applies in man, when they say that '. . . these results emphasize the necessity for caution in the interpretation of experiments done at low urine flows, or those in which urine is allowed to pool in the bladder during collection periods'.

It is also important to note that they showed diffusion of creatinine across the bladder wall and ureter. This is obviously a major problem for the standard method of correcting urine collections by expressing the results relative to creatinine excretion. It also raises the question as to how much of the 'diurnal' variation in GFR is due to creatinine reabsorption and water transfer.

It is obviously important to make a direct measurement of the permeability of the normal human bladder to creatinine. In theory, this is straightforward. It would require the instillation of normal saline into the bladder, leaving it there for say 60 min, and measuring the creatinine concentration. However, it also requires that there be no direct passage of urine into the bladder. Even in an institution such as ours, we have been unable to find a patient with a normal (i.e. nonaugmented, noninfected) bladder with diversion of the ureters. The experiment is obviously important, and we predict that the human bladder will be shown to be permeable to creatinine.

We suggest that all data based on bladder urinary concentration of solutes be regarded with caution.

References

1 Levinsky NG, Berliner RW; Changes in composition of the urine in ureter and bladder at low urine flow. Am J Physiol 1959;196:549–553.
2 Fellows GJ, Marshall DH: The permeability of human bladder epithelium to water and sodium. Invest Urol 1972;9:339–344.

A.J.W. Hilson, MB, MSc, FRCP, St. Paul's Hospital, Endell Street,
London WC2H 9AE (UK)

Blaufox MD, Hollenberg NK, Raynaud C (eds): Radionuclides in Nephro-Urology.
Contrib Nephrol. Basel, Karger, 1990, vol 79, pp 45–51

Prolonged Constant Dual-Isotope Infusion for Determination of Renal Function after Water Loading in Hypertensive Diabetic Men

K. Gish Herron, J. Folscroft, M. MacDougall, A. Chonko, T. Wiegmann

Department of Medicine, Division of Nephrology, University of Kansas Medical Center, and Nephrology Section, Medical Service, Department of Veterans Affairs, Kansas City, Mo., USA

Measurements of glomerular filtration rate (GFR) and effective renal plasma flow (RPF) with intravenous injections or constant infusions of radioactive tracers are well established. Radionuclides offer advantages over traditional inulin and PAH infusions because they can be detected and quantified easily and precisely in urine and plasma. Numerous investigations have shown high correlation between traditional methods and radionuclide tracers in clearance studies [1]. There is continued discussion, however, on the relative precision of different techniques. Some studies advocate the use of plasma disappearance data measured with one or more timed plasma samples [2–5]. Other investigators, studying patients with diabetes and other glomerular diseases, have favored the use of serial sampling of urine and plasma with either bolus injection or constant infusion of radioactive markers [6–8]. However, the clinical use of any clearance technique remains fraught with great variability between successive examinations in the same individual. This variability is most frequently attributed to problems in accurate collection of urine without catheters. This problem is of particular concern in patients who may not void predictably, for example, patients with diabetes mellitus, and these sampling problems may increase with progressive loss of renal function. In an effort to minimize errors from incomplete urine collections, water loading and intravenous hydration are done to ensure adequate diuresis. It is unknown, however, to what extent water loading may affect the renal functional response during determinations of GFR and RPF.

To examine the relationship between water loading and the determination of renal function by clearance methods, we have examined men with type II diabetes mellitus and hypertension. Standard water loading was used in combination with intravenous hydration to ensure diuresis. Con-

Table 1. Clinical characteristics (n = 55; mean ± SE)

Age	59.4 ± 1.1
Weight, kg	97.0 ± 3.0
Height, cm	176.8 ± 0.9
Surface, m^2	2.13 ± 0.04
BP systolic, mm Hg	149.9 ± 2.3
BP diastolic, mm Hg	88.5 ± 1.3

stant infusions of ^{125}I-iothalamate and ^{131}I-iodohippurate were used to determine GFR and RPF, respectively, in half-hour clearance intervals over 6 h. We also examined urine flow rates, solute and salt excretion. The studies reveal significant delay in the attainment of steady-state conditions and underscore the need to determine renal function after steady state is reached.

Materials and Methods

Participants in this study were recruited from an outpatient population and the clinical characteristics are given in table 1. Patients were included in the study if they had a proven diagnosis of type II diabetes mellitus and hypertension (n = 55). All patients gave informed consent. Thirty patients underwent a second study after entering a hypertension trial and these results were included in this study.

The patients were tested in the fasting state, thus insulin or oral hypoglycemic agents were withheld the morning of the study. Blood glucose concentration was maintained between 120 and 240 mg/dl. An indwelling intravenous catheter was placed in each arm, one for blood sampling (heparin lock) and the other for constant intravenous infusion. Patients remained in a sitting position for the duration of the study except for urination. An oral load of water (1% of BW, limit 1 liter) and an intravenous load of 0.45% NaCl (200 ml) were given initially. A urine and plasma sample were obtained 30–60 min after initiation of the water load where the precise timing was determined by the occurrence of spontaneous diuresis (collection 0). Complete voiding was encouraged by manual pressure over the bladder.

Radioactive tracers were added to the remaining intravenous solution (800 ml) for clearance determinations. ^{125}I-iothalamate (Iso-Tex Diagnostics, Inc., Austin, Tex.) clearance was taken to represent GFR while that of ^{131}I-iodohippurate (Squibb Pharmaceuticals, Princeton, N.J.) represented RPF. The total radioactive dose consisted of 80 μCi of ^{125}I-iothalamate and 200 μCi of ^{131}I-iodohippurate. An initial priming dose (25% of total) of this saline-isotope mixture (200 ml) was infused over the next 30 min (60–90 min from the start of the study). A mixture of 40,000 and 70,000 MW dextran solution (100 ml) was added during this time. After these infusions were complete, urine and plasma samples were obtained (collection 1). Altogether, at the end of collection period 1, the patient had received 400 ml of 0.45% NaCl, 100 ml of dextran and 10 ml/kg of oral water in a total time of 60–90 min. Continued diuresis was maintained by 100 ml of oral water and 50 ml of the saline isotope mixture every 30 min. Urine and plasma samples were collected every 30 min in the subsequent clearance periods (2–9). Occasionally, adjacent collection periods were combined during the early phases into a single collection because of inability to void.

Table 2. Excretion of solutes, GFR and RPF during water loading in patients with diabetes mellitus (85 studies)

Period	mosm/kg × min × 10^{-3}	GFR ml/min 1.73 m^2	RPF ml/min 1.73 m^2
1	6.0 ± 0.8	33.4 ± 3.2	350.1 ± 90.1
2	7.4 ± 0.8	76.2 ± 4.5	360.3 ± 28.3
3	6.3 ± 0.7	79.4 ± 4.3	356.4 ± 24.0
4	6.0 ± 0.6	76.2 ± 4.0	307.7 ± 16.2
5	5.5 ± 0.5	80.7 ± 5.7	297.1 ± 14.5
6	5.3 ± 0.5	74.4 ± 3.7	286.1 ± 12.9
7	5.0 ± 0.5	71.3 ± 3.5	282.7 ± 13.0
8	5.0 ± 0.5	71.7 ± 3.4	286.1 ± 12.0
9	5.0 ± 0.5	73.6 ± 4.0	277.8 ± 13.3

Total urinary solute (osmolar) concentration was determined by freezing-point depression and sodium was measured by flame photometry. Specific activity of ^{125}I-iothalamate and ^{131}I-iodohippurate in urine and plasma were determined by a Hewlett-Packard dual channel gamma scintillation spectrometer. Excretion of 'x' was determined from urinary concentration (U_x) and volume (V), while clearance was determined by the standard formula $U_x \times V/P_x \times T$, where P represents plasma concentration and *T* time in minutes. All results were corrected for 1.73 m^2 body surface. Analysis of variance was used for sequential samples while a t test was used for comparison of groups. A p value of < 0.05 was accepted as significant.

Results

Urine flow rates (ml/min) promptly increased after initial oral water loading and intravenous infusion. Normal daily urine flow rate (1–2) ml/min) was surpassed during period 1 (60–90 min after the beginning of the study). Mean urine flow rate exceeded 6 ml/min during period 3 and remained steady at this level throughout the remainder of the experiment. Plasma concentrations of each radionuclide reached a stable plateau at the end of period 2 (not shown).

Mean GFR during the early clearance phase (collections 2–5) was 78.1 ± 2.3 compared to 72.9 ± 7.8 ml/min 1.73 m^2 ($p < 0.1$) in the latter half of the experiment (collections 6–9). RPF was significantly higher during collection periods 2–5 (330.6 ± 10.9) compared to the latter half of the experiment (276.8 ± 6.3 ml/min 1.73 m^2; $p < 0.0001$; collection periods 6–9). These results were consistent with an initial increase in GFR and RPF due to the infusion and water load (table 2). We examined this perturbation more closely and also analyzed solute and salt excretion in all periods (table 2). Solute excretion peaked early (period 2), and then slowly

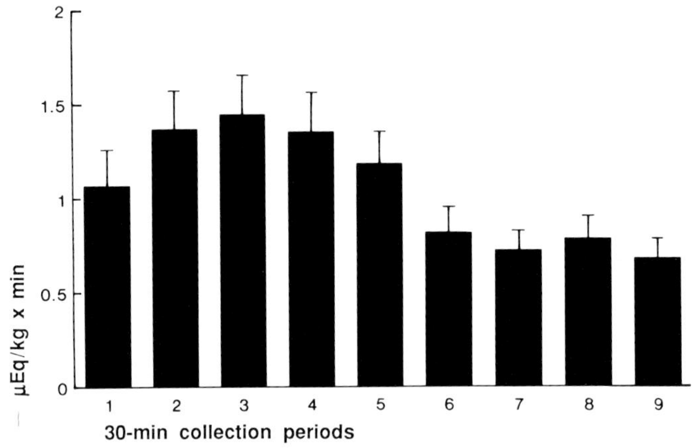

Fig. 1. Effect of water loading on urinary excretion of sodium in patients with diabetes mellitus (mean ± SE).

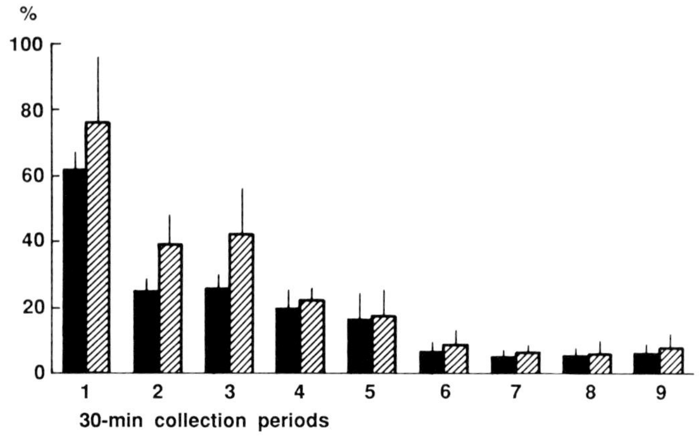

Fig. 2. Absolute difference (mean % ± SE) of individual clearance measurements from terminal average for GFR (■) and RPF (▨) in patients with diabetes mellitus.

approached a steady state. Sodium excretion peaked during period 3 and also slowly decreased toward a steady state (fig. 1).

Sodium and solute excretion data together with the difference between early and late results for GFR and RPF demonstrated a significant effect of water loading on renal function over a protracted period of time and a steady state was not achieved until the last four collection periods.

Therefore, individual measures of GFR and RPF were derived from the latter phases of the experiment by calculating the average of each patient's last four collection periods. Using these mean values for each patient, we then reevaluated each collection and their absolute differences from these means. The differences between single samples and the terminal mean was highest at the beginning of the experiment and lowest during steady state (fig. 2). These findings were similar when the data were reexamined separately for patients with a GFR of greater or less than 60 ml/min.

Discussion

This study demonstrates that the combination of water loading with small amounts of dilute electrolyte solution will lead to predictable and copious diuresis in patients with diabetes mellitus and hypertension. The protocol was well tolerated and resulted in timely spontaneous urination in most instances. Urine flow attained a steady state between 1 and 2 h after initiation of water loading. In contrast, there were significant differences in renal function over time. GFR and RPF as well as solute and salt excretion reached a predictable steady state 3–4 h after initiation of water loading. Successive determinations of GFR and RPF differed least during steady state.

Steady diuresis is an essential feature of renal function tests employing clearance techniques. Various methods are used to attain this diuresis, including oral water loading alone [6, 9], or with the addition of an electrolyte solution [8]. These protocols generally establish urine flow to a similar degree as the present study over a 1-hour period. We chose a combination of oral and intravenous hydration as some patients with diabetes mellitus may not initiate a prompt diuresis after oral hydration alone. This concern arises because such patients frequently exhibit delayed gastric emptying with consequent unpredictable water absorption.

Measurement of GFR and RPF was performed using a constant infusion technique with multiple clearance periods, similar to other studies in patients with diabetes [6, 7]. Ordinarily, clearance studies are performed immediately upon attainment of adequate urinary flow rate with only short additional periods (30–60 min) provided for the equilibration of tracer materials. Clearance studies are thus typically completed 3 h after initiation of water loading [6–8]. Such an observation period may be too short if a steady state has not been reached. A significant delay in the attainment of steady-state conditions for urinary solute and albumin excretion after oral water loading was found in previous renal function studies in patients with type I diabetes [unpubl. data]. We therefore extended the present study for up to 6 h. In this study, significant time-dependent differences were found for solute and salt excretion as well as GFR and RPF. Thus, a considerable amount of time elapsed before steady-state conditions were obtained. These effects were surprising because water intake is not thought to affect GFR and RPF and the total amount of electrolytes provided during initiation and maintenance of diuresis was small.

Many renal function studies have focused on different tracers or the relative merit of clearance techniques in comparison with plasma disappearance studies [7, 8]. Little attention has been paid to the effects of hydration on renal function and it is not clear whether previous studies were performed during steady state. It is therefore likely that comparisons between inulin or PAH and radioactive tracers develop similar results despite the fact that both may be affected by the lack of steady-state conditions. Under nonsteady-state conditions, one would not expect similarity of results between plasma disappearance and clearance results. For example, if terminal plasma data were seen as a global measure, unaffected by hydration, one would expect results to be smaller than early clearance measures. This could not be evaluated with constant infusions.

Based on urinary solute and salt excretion patterns in this study, we determined that the establishment of steady-state conditions was affected by hydration. Measures of renal function were higher during the early phases of the study, prior to reaching steady state. We attribute the variability between samples and the difference between early and late clearance periods to the physiologic effect of water loading. On the other hand, differences between collections during steady state are usually smaller and can be attributed to residual problems in obtaining reproducible urine collections without catheters. We suggest that clearance studies involving water loading must be performed after the achievement of steady-state conditions and that this does not usually occur until 4 h after water loading.

References

1 Chervu LR, Freeman LM, Blaufox MD: Radiopharmaceuticals for renal studies. Semin Nucl Med 1974;4:3–22.

2 Russell CD, Bischoff PG, Kontzen FN, et al: Measurement of glomerular filtration rate: single injection plasma clearance method without urine collection. J Nucl Med 1985;26:1243–1247.

3 Tauxe WN, Maher FT, Taylor WF: Effective renal plasma flow: Estimation from theoretical volumes of distribution of intravenously injected ^{131}I-orthoidodohippurate. Mayo Clin Proc 1971;46:524–531.

4 Blaufox MD, Merrill JP: Simplified hippuran clearance: Measurement of renal functions in man with simplified hippuran clearances. Nephron 1966;3:274–281.

5 Ram MD: A single injection method for measurement of effective renal plasma flow. Br J Urol 1968;40:425–428.
6 Mogensen CE: Glomerular filtration rate and renal plasma flow in short-term and long-term juvenile diabetes mellitus. Scand J Clin Lab Invest 1971;28:91–100.
7 Christiansen JS, Gammelgaard J, Frandsen M, et al: Increased kidney size, glomerular filtration rate and renal plasma flow in short-term insulin-dependent diabetics. Diabetologia 1981;20:451–456.
8 Shemesh O, Golbetz H, Kriss JP, et al: Limitations of creatinine as a filtration marker in glomerulopathic patients. Kidney Int 1985;28:830–838.
9 Adefuin PY, Gur A, Siegel NJ, et al: Single subcutaneous injection of iothalamate sodium I–125 to measure glomerular filtration rate. JAMA 1976;235:1467–1469.

T.B. Wiegmann, MD, VA Medical Center, Nephrology (111A),
4801 Linwood Boulevard, Kansas City, MO 64128 (USA)

Blaufox MD, Hollenberg NK, Raynaud C (eds): Radionuclides in Nephro-Urology.
Contrib Nephrol. Basel, Karger, 1990, vol 79, pp 52–57

Simultaneous Measurement of Glomerular Filtration Rate and Effective Renal Plasma Flow Reveals Increased Glomerular Capillary Pressure among Teenage Diabetic Subjects

E.P. Paulsen, F.L. Pauly, B.Y. Croft, C.D. Teates

Departments of Pediatrics and Radiology, University of Virginia Health Sciences Center, Charlottesville, Va., USA

Two hypotheses have been suggested to explain the etiology of diabetic nephropathy which occurs in 33–40% of youth-onset insulin-dependent diabetic subjects [1]. One suggests that sustained increases in glomerular flow and pressure which accompany hyperglycemia are the initiating factors [2]. However, the statistics defining risk for nephropathy as occurring in a third of diabetic subjects were gathered before strict glycemic control was achievable in any significant percentage of diabetics. The other hypothesis suggests that mesangial expansion coupled with decreased filtering surface leads to functional glomerular deterioration [3]. The hypothesis does not define a mechanism which initiates mesangial expansion in a select one-third of diabetics destined to develop nephropathy.

Reports of high plasma renin activity among teenage and young adult [4] insulin-dependent diabetic subjects suggested that associated increases in angiotensin II production could lead to increased intrarenal pressure and be the initiating factor in mesangial expansion, appearance of albuminuria, and, over time, of cell death and glomerular sclerosis. Resting and stimulated levels of plasma renin activity were, therefore, measured in a cohort of early pubertal, adolescent, and young adult diabetic subjects in whom insulin dependency was certain [5]. Simultaneous measurement of glomerular filtration rate GFR and effective renal plasma flow (ERPF) were carried out to determine glomerular capillary pressure as reflected in renal vascular resistance. Glomerular capillary pressure is significantly affected by renin-induced angiotension II production in the kidney [6].

Materials and Methods

Sixty subjects (28 females and 32 males) 13–30 years of age, diagnosed with insulin-dependent diabetes (type 1) before age 16, were admitted to the Clinical Research Center for study. They are part of a cohort of 100 subjects assessed between 13 and 20 years of age who have undergone serial studies for a maximum of 4.6 ± 0.2 (SEM) years. During the admission, diet consisted of 50% carbohydrate, 15% protein, 35% fat (polyunsaturated:saturated: 1.5:1.0) with restriction of refined sugar and caffeinated beverages, salt according to taste, and no restriction of caloric or fluid intake.

GFR, using ^{99m}Tc-DTPA and ERPF, using ^{131}I-hippuran, were measured simultaneously with the subject in the supine resting position. The single-injection, multiple blood-sampling technique was used. Blood was sampled at 5, 10, 15, 20, 25, 30, 40, 50, 60, 70, 80 and 90 min postinjection. Three-milliliter blood samples were counted in a multichannel well counter and compared with a set of standards. The ^{99m}Tc counts were corrected for decay during the counting process. A computer program did log-linear least squares fits of the data to a biexponential curve. The results were checked by the operator and the processing corrected when obviously spurious results were obtained.

Measurements of GFR, but not ERPF, and a simultaneous HbA_1 were made in an additional 40 diabetic subjects in the same age range as the cohort of 60 and are utilized in obtaining the associations given in figure 1.

Filtration fraction (FF) was derived by dividing GFR by ERPF. Renal vascular resistance (RVR) was calculated by dividing mean arterial pressure (MAP) by renal blood flow (RBF = [ERPF/0.9]/[1 – HCT]).

GFR and ERPF data were interpreted in terms of urinary microalbumin or protein excretion resting and stimulated plasma renin activity (PRA), and glycemic control (HbA_1) [5]. The subjects are separated into four groups based on microalbumin excretion rates (AER), a predictor of clinical nephropathy in insulin-dependent diabetic subjects (IDDS): group 1 (50%) – normal AER at rest and during exercise; group 2 (28%) – normal AER at rest but abnormally elevated during exercise; group 3 (14%) – abnormally elevated AER at rest and during exercise, and group 4 (8%) – fixed clinical proteinuria unchanged at rest and during exercise.

All subjects and parents of those under 18 years of age were informed of the nature and purpose of the tests before giving consent to participate. Tests were approved by the Human Investigation Committee of the University of Virginia Medical Center.

Statistical analyses were performed using Student's t statistic and regression analyses. All values are mean ± SEM unless otherwise designated.

Results

The number of subjects in each AER group (table 1) are proportional to those in the cohort of 100 under study [5]. IDDS with abnormal AER at rest and during exercise (group 3) or with fixed clinical proteinuria (group 4) are significantly older than those with normal AER (group 1) or with abnormal AER during exercise (group 2). Glycemic control (HbA_1) is similar among the four groups. Renal function reflected in serum levels of BUN and creatinine is normal in AER group 1–3 but mildly abnormal in group 4.

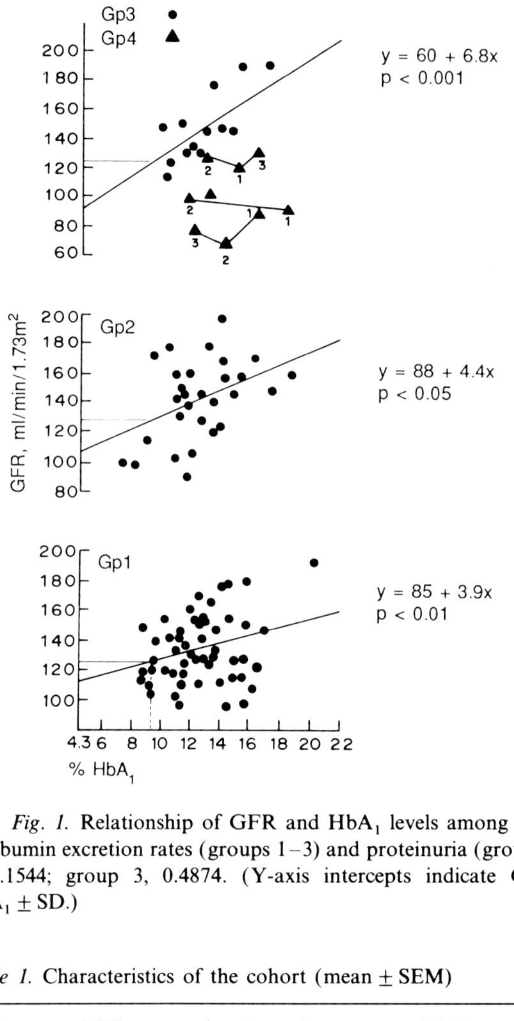

Fig. 1. Relationship of GFR and HbA_1 levels among 100 IDDS grouped on the basis of albumin excretion rates (groups 1–3) and proteinuria (group 4). R^2: group 1, 0.1578; group 2, 0.1544; group 3, 0.4874. (Y-axis intercepts indicate GFR corresponding to normal $HbA_1 \pm SD$.)

Table 1. Characteristics of the cohort (mean ± SEM)

AER group	F/M n	Age (range) years	BUN mg/dl	Cr_s mg/dl	HbA_1 %
1	16/16	21 ± 1 (13–30)	14 ± 0.5	0.8 ± 0.02	13.4 ± 0.5
2	8/8	21 ± 1 (15–29)	14 ± 0.5	0.9 ± 0.04	12.2 ± 0.6
3	2/5	24 ± 2[a] (15–28)	13 ± 1.6	0.9 ± 0.03	11.1 ± 0.5
4	2/3	24 ± 1[a] (21–26)	20 ± 2[b]	1.6 ± 0.19[c]	13.6 ± 1.0
Normal values			10 – 20	0.7 – 1.3	6.9 ± 0.1

p values 3, 4 vs. 1, 2 < [a]0.02, [b]0.001, [c]0.0001.

Table 2. Functional parameters based on albumin excretion rates (mean ± SEM)

AER group	GFR ml/min/ 1.73 m^2	ERPF	MAP, mm Hg female	MAP, mm Hg male	FF	RVR 10^3 dyn·s·cm^5/ m^2
1	148 ± 4^d	631 ± 18^d	79 ± 2	83 ± 1	0.24 ± 0.01^d	5.7 ± 0.2
2	150 ± 4^d	628 ± 31^b	81 ± 3	84 ± 2	0.24 ± 0.01^d	5.7 ± 0.3
3	139 ± 7^c	538 ± 34	86 ± 1^b	92 ± 2^c	0.26 ± 0.02^d	7.2 ± 0.5^b
4	69 ± 12^a	350 ± 32^c	90 ± 1^a	111 ± 3^c	0.20	12.9 ± 1.9^d
Normal values	111 ± 3	553 ± 20	79 ± 1	84 ± 3	0.16 ± 0.20	6.2 ± 0.2

p values versus normal: < [a]0.05, [b]0.01, [c]0.001, [d]0.0001.

GFR and ERPF are markedly elevated in AER groups 1 and 2 (table 2). GFR remains elevated in group 3 but ERPF is significantly reduced. Both functions are abnormally low in group 4. FF is elevated in groups 1–3. MAP and RVR are normal in groups 1 and 2, abnormal in group 3, and markedly so in group 4.

Significant associations are noted among measured functions (GFR, MAP, AER, PRA, HbA_1) and derived functions (FF, RVR): *RVR* with FF ($p < 0.001$) and with PRA ($p < 0.02$) but not with GFR or HbA_1; *AER at rest* with MAP ($p < 0.01$), and with RVR ($p < 0.001$) but not with HbA_1; *AER during exercise* with MAP ($p < 0.01$), and with RVR ($p < 0.02$), and HbA_1 ($p < 0.001$); *GFR in groups 1–3*, not group 4, with HbA_1 (fig. 1). Mean GRF and intercepts on the y-axis for the normal $HbA_1 \pm 2$ SD (4.3–9.5%) are normal and similar in groups 1 and 2; 118 ± 4, 110–126; 118 ± 5, 108–128 ml/min/1.73 m^2. The values are significantly lower in group 3 when compared to those in groups 1 and 2: 108 ± 7, 92–123, $p < 0.001$.

Discussion

The transition from normal AER or abnormal AER during exercise to abnormal AER during rest and exercise or clinical proteinuria is paralleled by an increase in age, decreases in renal plasma flow, increases in MAP, and marked advances in RVR. The association of increased RVR with high FF is consistent with postglomerular constriction and increased glomerular capillary pressure. The association of RVR and PRA suggests that angiotensin II, generated by renin action, underlies the increased pressure.

Angiotensin II acts preferentially on mesangial cells and efferent arterioles; both are highly sensitive to its vasoconstrictive action [6]. The exaggerated levels of angiotensin II could, together with the high prevailing renal plasma flow rates, enhance capillary pressure, and, under appropriate conditions described below, initiate AER.

The observation that abnormal microalbuminuria first appears during exercise suggests that metabolic and pressure changes associated with exercise in the susceptible diabetic subject play important roles. During exercise, increases in plasma catecholamines, renin activity, and lactate parallel the intensity of work. Subjects liberating the most lactate have the highest increases in PRA. Strenuous exercise in diabetic subjects results in higher lactate levels than in normal subjects [7].

The initial appearance of abnormal microalbuminuria in puberty [5] suggests that hormonal changes play a role. In healthy young menstruating females, capillary permeability to protein and water measured by venous occlusion of the forearm in enhanced in the luteal phase compared with the estrogen phase [8] and PRA is increased during the luteal phase of the normal menstrual cycle.

Insulin plays a role in reducing glomerular capillary permeability to albumin by stimulating synthesis of sialic acid and proteoglycans in the basement membrane. These negatively charged polyanions which repel macromolecules of like charge, such as plasma albumin, are markedly decreased in renal tissue of diabetic humans [9] and streptozotocin-treated mice and are restored to normal by insulin treatment. The significant association between increased AER during exercise and HbA_1 levels in groups 2 and 3 supports a role for insulin in reducing glomerular permeability in these subjects. However, absence of an association between HbA_1 and abnormal AER at rest, as well as the presence of elevated HbA_1 in some subjects of AER group 1, indicates that adequate insulinization is not the primary factor in the appearance of abnormal AER. The lack of an association between HbA_1 and RVR or MAP suggests that improved glycemic control, though it may reduce albumin excretion, does not affect glomerular capillary pressure.

GRF is significantly increased in newly diagnosed or poorly controlled diabetic subjects [10]. In the present study, GFR reached equally high levels in subjects with normal or with abnormal AER, suggesting that elevated GFR does not initiate abnormal AER. Continued exposure of glomeruli to increased flow and pressure, the two major determinants of GFR, may, in the context of heightened RVR, contribute to the progression of clinical nephropathy.

The significant association between GFR and HbA_1 in this study indicates a role for insulin in maintaining normal GFR noted by others, but the underlying mechanism continues to elude discovery. Regression analysis permits calculation of true GFR and reveals a minimal but significant decline in GFR among subjects of group 3.

References

1 Knowles HC, Guest GM, Lampe J, et al: The course of juvenile diabetes treated with unmeasured diet. Diabetes 1965;14:239–273.
2 Hostetter TH, Renneke HG, Brenner BM: The case for intrarenal hypertension in the initiation and progression of diabetic and other glomerulopathies. Am J Med 1982;72:375–380.
3 Mauer SM, Steffes MW, Ellis EN, et al: Structural-functional relationships in diabetic nephropathy. J Clin Invest 1984;74:1143–1155.
4 Gossain VV, Werk EE, Sholiton LJ, et al: Plasma renin activity in juvenile diabetes mellitus and effect of diazoxide. Diabetes 1975;24:833–835.
5 Paulsen EP, Seip RL, Ayers CR, et al: Plasma renin activity and albumin excretion in teenage type I diabetic subjects: a prospective study. Hypertension 1989 13;781–788.
6 Navar LG, Rosival L: Contribution of the renin-angiotensin system to the control of intrarenal hemodynamics. Kidney Int 1984;25:857–868.
7 Berger M, Berchthold P, Cuppers HJ, et al: Metabolic and hormonal effects of muscular exercise in juvenile type diabetics. Diabetologia 1977;13:355–365.
8 Mahajan KK, Marya RK, Maini BK, et al: Capillary permeability during the menstrual cycle. Indian J Med 1973;27:693–696.
9 Westburg NG, Michael AF: Human glomerular basement membrane: clinical composition in diabetes mellitus. Acta Med Scand 1973;194:39–47.
10 Christiansen JS, Gammelgaard J, Grandsen M, et al: Increased kidney size, glomerular filtration rate and renal plasma flow in short-term insulin-dependent diabetics. Diabetologia 1981;20:451–456.

Dr. E.P. Paulsen, Department of Pediatrics, Box 386,
University of Virginia Medical Center, Charlottesville, VA 22908 (USA)

Blaufox MD, Hollenberg NK, Raynaud C (eds): Radionuclides in Nephro-Urology. Contrib Nephrol. Basel, Karger, 1990, vol 79, pp 58–62

Clinical Evaluation of the Filtration Fraction: Multivariate Statistical Analysis

W.N. Tauxe[a], *D. Kundu*[b], *H.A. Klein*[a]

[a]Division of Nuclear Medicine and [b]Department of Mathematics and Statistics, University of Pittsburgh, Pa., USA

The filtration fraction (FF), as a concept to represent that portion of the total effective renal plasma flow (ERPF) filtered by the glomerulus as the glomerular filtration rate (GFR), was mentioned by Smith [1] as early as 1938. Since this publication, numerous other references have appeared [e.g., 2, 3], but few have evaluated its clinical use.

We have studied the FF in normal kidney donors before and after nephrectomy, in hypertensive patients and in kidney recipients. The purpose of this paper is to present the results of that evaluation.

Materials and Methods

Selection of subjects: To observe the general relationship between GFR and ERPF, 134 studies in 74 consecutive patients referred to the nuclear medicine service for renal function evaluation were chosen for study. GFR and ERPF determinations were carried out simultaneously by single injection techniques described previously [4, 5]. FF was calculated as the quotient GFR/ERPF.

From this mixed group, subjects in the following categories were chosen for this study: normal subjects before (9) and after (14) kidney donation; normally functioning kidney recipients (35); chronically rejecting recipients (5), recipients with cell-mediated rejection (2), renovascular hypertension (13), essential hypertension (21), malignant hypertension (2).

Since the data from the groups overlapped, a special analysis by method of elliptical confidence regions (ECR) was developed. Clustering of various clinical groups was sought on FF-ERPF data. We assumed the underlying distribution to be a multivariate normal, whose density is given by: $f(x) = C_p|\Sigma|^{-\frac{1}{2}} \exp[\frac{1}{2}(\mathbf{x}-\boldsymbol{\mu})'\Sigma^{-1}(\mathbf{x}-\boldsymbol{\mu})]$, where C_p is a constant, $\boldsymbol{\mu}$ = a $p \times 1$ mean vector and Σ is the $p \times p$ covariance matrix for the p-variate x; therefore, we have not assumed independence between the variables. So all sample observations (here 2-vectors) from k-th group were assumed to be independently and identically distributed as normal distribution with main vector μ_k and common variance-covariance matrix Σ.

To test whether group i and group j could be clustered together amounted to testing the null hypothesis: $\mu i = \mu j$ against the alternative: $\mu i \neq \mu j$. This problem was put into the framework of general linear model and multiple comparison of mean vectors were made. We

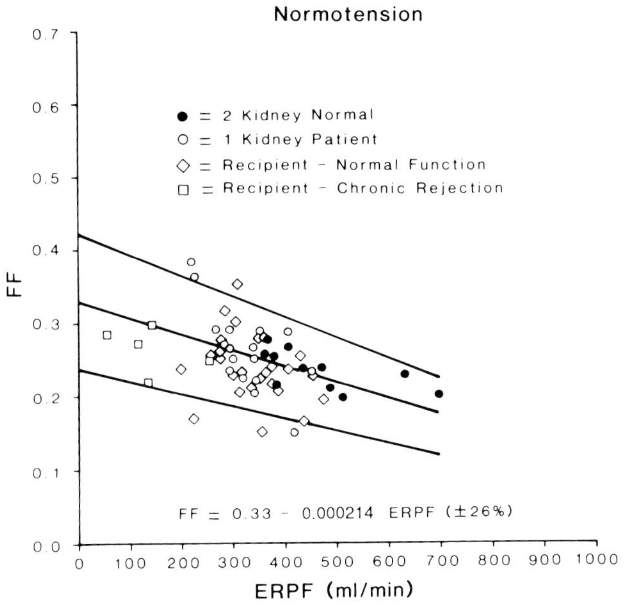

Fig. 1. Plot of FF against ERPF in all cases in series involved with renal transplantation, donors and recipients. Two SD are shown. There is an apparent continuum of normal two kidneyed patients below the line starting on the right through one kidneyed normal adults, normally functioning transplants, rejecting patients on the left.

applied Krishnaiah's finite intersection tests (FIT) [6] for multiple comparison for the data analysis. The computer program for implementation of FIT was described by Cox et al. [7].

For each significantly different group we used Hotelling T^2 statistic to find the 99%-confidence regions for the respective population mean vector around the sample mean as the set of all points (2-vector) satisfying $(y - \mu)\, S^{-1}\, (y - \mu) < C_\alpha$ where, y = sample mean vector for the related group, S = sample variance-covariance matrix

$$C_\alpha = \frac{p(n-1)}{n(n-p)} F_\alpha, \quad \text{for } \alpha = 0.01,\ p = 2$$

n = number of sample points from the group and F_α = percentile point from the F-distribution with degrees of freedom (p, n-p).

These confidence sets were ellipses with length of the semi-major and semi-minor axes proportional to the square root of the largest two eigenvalues of S.

Results

When all FF values are plotted against ERPF, errors are particularly high at the lower end of the scale where GFR and ERPF values are low

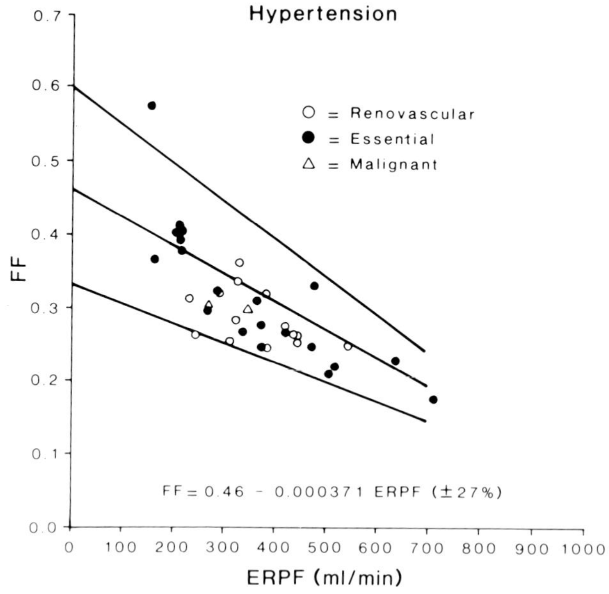

Fig. 2. Plot of FF against ERPF in all hypertensive cases. Most FF lie above and roughly parallel to the regression line shown in figure 1. No clustering among diagnostic categories was found.

and errors of measurement of each variable are relatively high. The best fitting regression line through all the data indicate that FF is a function of ERPF. The formula for the regression line is: FF = 0.377–0.000314 ERPF. Using the ECR method, significant differences were observed among three groups: (A) normal donor subjects with two kidneys; (B) subjects with a single kidney (fig.1), and (C) hypertensive patients, at a significance level of $\alpha = < 0.001$.

FF from all hypertensive patients formed an identifiable group (fig. 2). Their FF values fell along but above the regression line of the whole population.

The 99% confidence ellipses for means of the three groups are depicted in fig. 3. Coefficients for these ellipses are: normal (2 kidney) $x' = 485.7$, $y' = 0.227$, $a = 0.000117$, $b = 0.3097$, $c = 2498.087$, $d = 2.4254$ hypertensives $x' = 355.2$, $y' = 0.304$, $a = 0.000142$, $b = 0.1895$, $c = 434.2469$, $d = 0.3037$; one kidney $x' = 314.2$, $y' = 0.262$, $a = 0.000642$, $b = 0.4372$, $c = 569{,}301.6$, $d = 1.0725$. These are based on FF-ERPF data in the form: $a(x - x')^2 + 2b(x - x')(y - y') + c(y - y')^2 \leqslant d$.

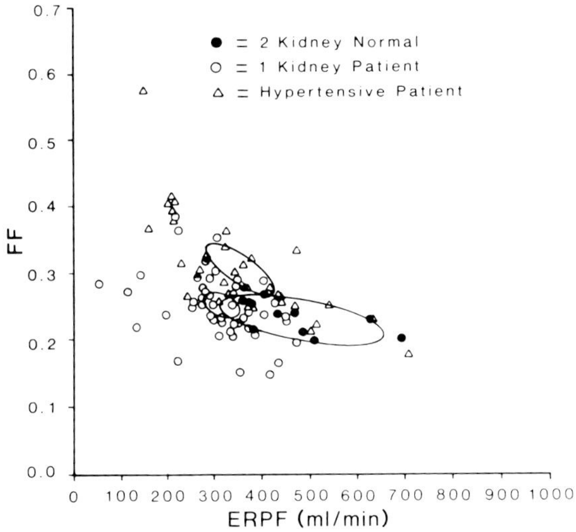

Fig. 3. Plot of data from normal (one kidney and two kidney), transplanted and hypertensive groups. Ellipses represent 99% confidence limits of locus of centroid of the groups. Although a small overlap between confidence limits in subjects with two and one kidneys is observed, the differences are significant.

Discussion

That FF increases as ERPF is diminished as by removal of a normal kidney was reported in 1974 by Skov and Hansen [8]. They attributed the fact to a 'change in hemodynamic pattern, affecting afferent and efferent arterioles provided that membrane characteristics are unchanged' rather than changes in hydration, blood pressure, weight, or circulatory status. This FF/ERPF negative regression line suggests that the concept of a normal free-standing GFR is not tenable, without taking the ERPF into consideration. Just why the FF increases as ERPF decreases is still not clear. The phenomenon has led to the concept of the 'hyperfiltering glomerulus' [9].

The statistical methods employed here have proven to be especially useful in processing group data of this form. A complete discussion of the merits of FIT over other multiple comparison test procedures is given by Cox et al. [10].

References

1 Smith HW, Goldring W, Chasis H: The measurement of the tubular excretory mass, effective blood flow and filtration rate in the normal human kidney. J Clin Invest 1938;17:263–278.

2 Cutler RE, Glatte H: Simultaneous measurement of glomerular filtration rate and effective renal plasma flow with ^{57}Co-cyancobalamine and ^{131}I-hippuran. J Lab Clin Med 1965;65:1041–1046.

3 Bianchi C, Bonadio M, Donadio C, et al: Filtration Fraction in Unilateral Hypertensive Renal Disease and a New Noninvasive Method for Its Measurement. Contrib. Nephrol. Basel, Karger, 1978, vol. 11, pp 29–49.

4 Wagoner RD, Tauxe WN, Maher FT, et al: Measurement of effective renal plasma flow with sodium iodohippurate ^{131}I. JAMA 1964;187:811–813.

5 Farmer CD, Tauxe WN, Maher FT, et al: Measurement of renal function with radioiodinated diatrizoate and *O*-iodohippurate. Am J Clin Pathol. 1967;47:9–16.

6 Krishnaiah PR: Multiple comparison tests in multiresponse experiments. Sankhya (Ser A) 1965;27:65–72.

7 Cox CM, Fang C, Boudreau RM: Computer program for Krishnaiah's finite intersection tests for multiple comparisons of mean vectors, unpubl. tech. rep. No 81–2, University of Pittsburgh.

8 Skov PE, Hansen HE: Glomerular filtration rate, renal plasma flow and filtration fraction in living donors before and after nephrectomy. Acta Med Scand 1974;195:97–103.

9 Hostetter TH: The hyperfiltering glomerulus. Med Clin N Am 1984;68:387–398.

10 Cox CM, Krishnaiah PR, Lee JC, et al: A study on finite intersection tests for multiple comparisons of means; in Krishnaiah PR (ed): International Symposium on Multivariate Analysis. Amsterdam, N.Y., North-Holland, 1978, vol 5.

W. Newlon Tauxe, MD, Divisions of Nuclear Medicine,
Presbyterian-University Hospital, Room 4880, Main Tower,
DeSoto at O'Hara Streets, Pittsburgh, PA 15213 (USA)

Blaufox MD, Hollenberg NK, Raynaud C (eds): Radionuclides in Nephro-Urology.
Contrib Nephrol. Basel, Karger, 1990, vol 79, pp 63–67

Renal Tubular Reabsorption of Calcium in Primary Hyperparathyroidism

J.H. Kristiansen[a], *J. Brøchner-Mortensen*[b], *K.O. Pedersen*[c], *S. Jensen*[a], *T. Glud*[d]

Departments of [a]Medicine and Endocrinology, [b]Clinical Physiology, [c]Clinical Chemistry, and [d]Medicine and Nephrology, Aalborg Hospital, Aalborg, Denmark

As an extension of our recent study of familial hypocalciuric hypercalcaemia (FHH) [1] we investigated the renal tubular handling of calcium in patients with primary hyperparathyroidism (PHPT) by means of simultaneous determination of the glomerular filtration rate (GFR) and the renal plasma clearance of lithium (Cl_{Li}).

Methods

Nine patients with PHPT (6 premenopausal, 2 postmenopausal females, and 1 male aged 38–66 years, mean 49 years) were investigated. Nine age-, sex- and surface-matched healthy volunteers formed a control group.

All measurements of calcium were made after an overnight fast on urine collected between 08.00–10.00 and 10.00–11.30 h and serum samples obtained at 08.30, 10.00 and 11.30 h. During the previous evening all subjects were given 16.2 mmol of lithium as Li_2Co_3, and until the examination was completed no methylxanthine-containing beverages were allowed. Biochemical analyses and clearance measurements were made by conventional laboratory techniques. GFR was determined from the renal plasma clearance of ^{51}Cr[EDTA]. Serum immunoreactive parathyroid hormone (S-iPTH) was determined by a two-site immunoradiometric assay [2].

The relationship between filtered and excreted calcium was constructed for the normal controls by a method described elsewhere [1]. The total absolute tubular reabsorption rate of calcium related to GFR (Tub_{Ca}/GFR) was determined as the difference between the ultrafiltrable serum calcium and the urinary excretion rate of calcium related to GFR. The proximal fractional reabsorption rate of calcium was determined as 1-Cl_{Li}/GFR. The proximal absolute reabsorption rate of calcium was determined in relation to GFR as the ultrafiltrable serum calcium multiplied with 1-Cl_{Li}/GFR. The distal tubular fractional reabsorption rate of calcium was determined as 1-Cl_{Ca}/Cl_{Li}, where Cl_{Ca} is the renal plasma clearance of calcium. The distal absolute reabsorption rate of calcium was determined in relation to GFR as the difference between total reabsorption rate and proximal reabsorption rate of calcium.

Table 1. Serum, urine, clearance and tubular reabsorption values (mean ± SD) in PHPT patients and controls

	$S\text{-}Ca^{++}$ mmol/l	$S\text{-}Uf_{Ca}$ mmol/l	U_{Ca} mmol/h	S-iPTH ng/l	GFR ml/min	Cl_{Li} ml/min	PFR_{Ca} %	PAR_{Ca}/GFR mmol/l	DFR_{Ca} %	DAR_{Ca}/GFR mmol/l
Patients (n = 9)	1.56 ±0.11***	1.71 ±0.12***	0.24 ±0.07***	119 ±29***	80.4 ±14.8*	19.5 ±4.4	75.8 ±3.7	1.30 ±0.10***	87.6 ±5.6**	0.37 ±0.07*
Controls (n = 9)	1.29 ±0.04	1.41 ±0.08	0.12 ±0.04	30 ±9	96.1 ±12.4	21.6 ±2.8	77.3 ±3.3	1.09 ±0.08	93.1 ±2.6	0.30 ±0.05

$S\text{-}Ca^{++}$ = Ionized serum calcium; $S\text{-}Uf_{Ca}$ = ultrafiltrable serum calcium; U_{Ca} = urinary calcium excretion rate; S-iPTH = serum immunoreactive parathyroid hormone; PFR_{Ca} = proximal fractional reabsorption; PAR_{Ca}/GFR = proximal absolute reabsorption; DFR_{Ca} = distal fractional reabsorption; DAR_{Ca}/GFR = distal absolute reabsorption.
Significance of difference from controls: $^{*}p < 0.05$; $^{**}p < 0.02$; $^{***}p < 0.01$.

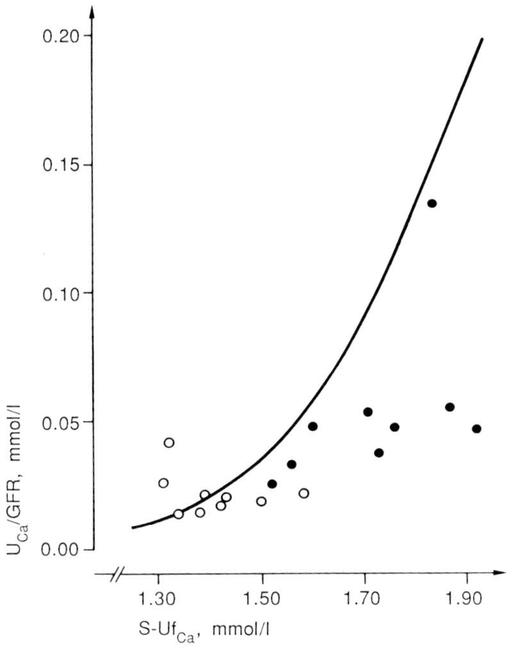

Fig. 1. The relation between ultrafiltrable and excreted calcium in normal controls (○) and PHPT patients (●).

Serum and urinary calcium data from PHPT patients were plotted in relation to the graph (fig. 1), and the increased capacity for tubular calcium reabsorption in each of the PHPT patients was determined as $100 \times (Tub_{Ca}/GFR$-'Tub_{Ca}/GFR')/'Tub_{Ca}/GFR', where 'Tub_{Ca} GFR' is the tubular reabsorption, if the PHPT patient had had a normal capacity, and was estimated for each PHPT patient as the difference between the ultrafiltrable serum calcium concentration and the urinary calcium excretion rate, which corresponds to the point of intersection between the graph (fig. 1) and a vertical line through the ultrafiltrable serum calcium value concerned.

Results

Serum and urinary calcium values and S-iPTH were significantly higher in PHPT patients than in normal controls (table 1). Figure 1 shows that corresponding serum and urinary calcium values from all cases with PHPT fall below and to the right of the normal relationship, indicating an increased capacity for renal tubular reabsorption of calcium.

In the proximal as well in the distal tubule there was a significantly higher absolute reabsorption rate of calcium in the PHPT group, whereas the fractional reabsorption rate of calcium in proximal tubule did not differ

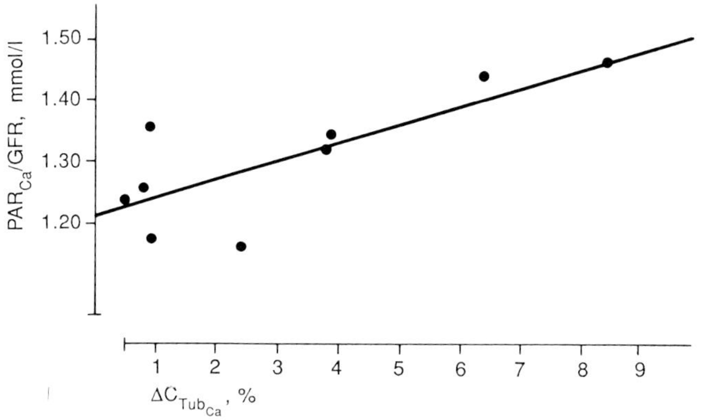

Fig. 2. The relationship between the increased capacity for tubular reabsorption of calcium ($C_{Tub_{Ca}}$) and the absolute reabsorption of calcium in the proximal tubule (PAR_{Ca}/GFR) in PHPT patients ($r = 0.77$, $p < 0.02$, $y = 0.0304x + 1.2095$).

between the two study groups, and the fractional reabsorption rate of calcium in the distal tubule was significantly lower in PHPT patients (table 1). There was a significantly positive correlation between the increased capacity for tubular reabsorption of calcium and the proximal absolute reabsorption rate related to GFR (fig. 2).

Discussion

The present results have shown an increased urinary excretion rate of calcium in PHPT compared with normal controls. This is a well-known feature of PHPT as it reflects the enhancing effect of PTH on calcium flux from gut and bone into the extracellular volume [3, 4].

The increased absolute tubular reabsorption of calcium seems to take place in the proximal as well as in the distal tubules. The increased calcium reabsorption in the proximal tubule may not be accounted for in full by the increased filtered load of calcium, since the relationship demonstrated in figure 2 suggests an existence of increased capacity for tubular calcium reabsorption in proximal tubules. This means that the proximal calcium reabsorption is higher in PHPT than in subjects with the same elevated ultrafiltrable calcium concentration, but with normal capacity. The lack of a significant correlation between the increased capacity and the absolute distal calcium reabsorption might suggest that the increased capacity for tubular calcium reabsorption is attached mainly to the proximal tubule.

Our recently published results about FHH [4] also suggested an increased capacity for calcium reabsorption in the proximal tubule but otherwise aspects of the pathophysiology differ between FHH and PHPT in that neither the urinary calcium excretion rate nor the distal tubular reabsorption of calcium differed between FHH and normal controls.

References

1 Kristiansen JH, Brøchner-Mortensen J, Pedersen KO: Renal tubular reabsorption of calcium in familial hypocalciuric hypercalcaemia. Acta Endocrinol 1986;112:541–546.

2 Nussbaum SR, Zahradnik RJ, Lavigne JR, et al: Highly sensitive two-site immunoradiometric assay of parathyrin, and its clinical utility in evaluating patients with hypercalcemia. Clin Chem 1987;33:1364–1368.

3 Nordin BEC, Horsmann A, Aaron J: Diagnostic procedures; in Nordin BEC (ed): Calcium, Phosphate and Magnesium Metabolism. Edinburgh, Churchill Livingstone, 1976, pp 469–525.

4 Charles P, Mosekilde L, Taagehøj-Jensen F: Primary hyperparathyroidism: evaluated by calcium-47 kinetics, calcium balance and serum bone-Gla-protein. Eur J Clin Invest 1986;16:277–283.

J.H. Kristiansen, MD, Department of Medicine and Endocrinology,
Aalborg Hospital, DK–9000 Aalborg (Denmark)

Blaufox MD, Hollenberg NK, Raynaud C (eds): Radionuclides in Nephro-Urology.
Contrib Nephrol. Basel, Karger, 1990, vol 79, pp 68–71

Renal Parenchymal Transit Time of $^{99m}Tc-MAG_3$ from Factor Analysis and from Region-of-Interest Selection in Hydronephrosis

C.D. Russell, M.V. Yester, E.V. Dubovsky
Division of Nuclear Medicine, University of Alabama Hospital, Birmingham, Ala., USA

Because of thinned cortex and marked pelvic retention, it is difficult to obtain parenchymal time-activity curves free of cross-talk from the pelvis in hydronephrotic kidneys. Verboven et al. [1] recently reported that measurement of mean parenchymal transit time (MPTT) was of little help in determining whether hydronephrotic kidneys had significant obstruction. Factor analysis, in theory, permits separation of time-activity curves even from spatially overlapping organs. $^{99m}Tc-MAG_3$, because of its high renal uptake and good statistics, lends itself to this approach. Here we report preliminary findings in a small group of patients.

Methods

Factor analysis was performed using Barber's method [2] with two modifications: (1) interpolative background subtraction (to eliminate the background factor) and (2) allowing the pelvic factor to lie outside the vertex of the factor polyhedron when necessary to achieve an initial slope of zero for the pelvic time-activity curve (corresponding to nephron transit). Operator intervention was required only to designate a rectangular region-of-interest (ROI) including the kidney. Three measures of parenchymal transit were used, two from the factor curves and one from a 2-pixel-wide cortical ROI: MPTT from deconvolution of the cortical factor time-activity curve (either ROI or factor) using the modified Kuruc method [3], or pelvic appearance time defined as the time when the pelvic factor curve reached half the maximum value attained in the first 20 frames (6.7 min). The patient population included 11 normal kidneys, 6 hydronephrotic kidneys with lack of significant obstruction demonstrated either by diuretic renography or by stable function for 12 months or longer, and 4 kidneys with significant obstruction demonstrated either by diuretic renography or deterioration in function.

Results

Figures 1 and 2 show factor images and curves for a normal kidney. Figure 1 also includes for comparison two other functional images that are

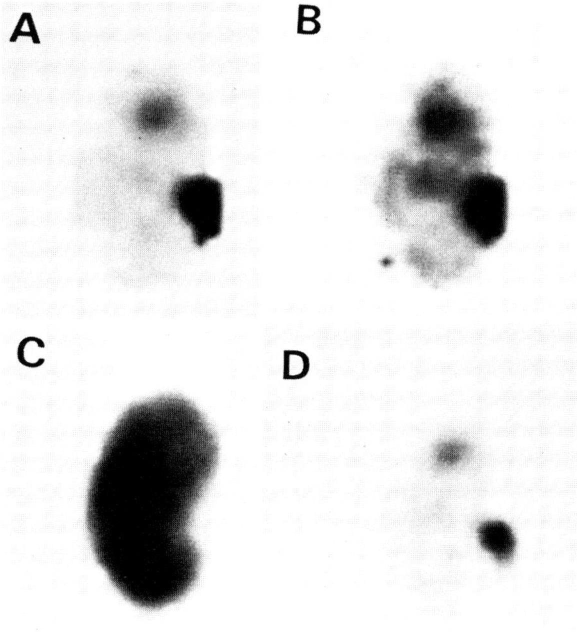

Fig. 1. Functional images obtained with $^{99m}Tc-MAG_3$ for a normal transplanted kidney. *A* First moment. *B* Peak time. *C* Cortical factor. *D* Pelvic factor.

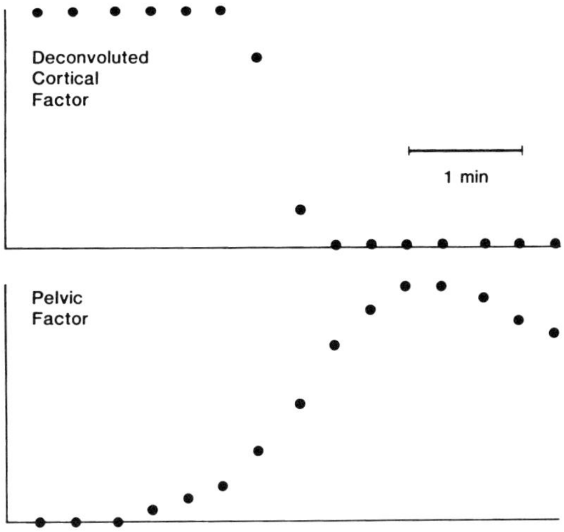

Fig. 2. Factor curves from normal kidney. Top: deconvoluted cortical factor; bottom: pelvic factor.

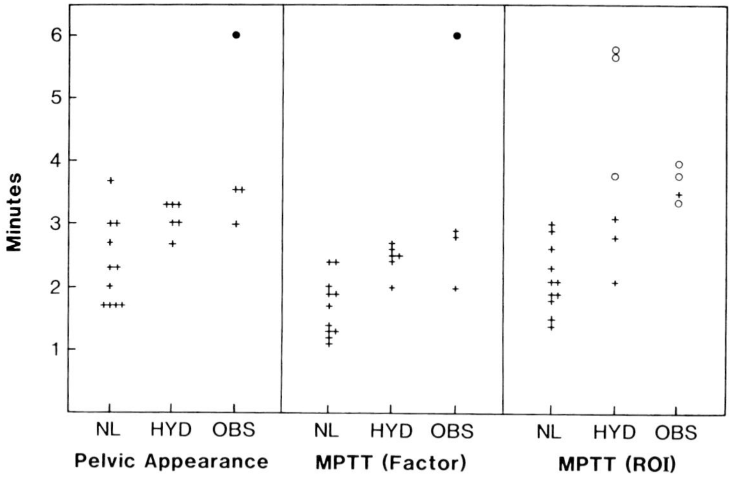

Fig. 3. Parenchymal transit times by three methods in normal, hydronephrotic but unobstructed, and obstructed kidneys. Solid circles: no activity seen in pelvis; open circles: transit not complete at 6.7 min; mean transit time is greater than plotted value.

commonly used to separate cortex from pelvis: a peak time image and a first-moment (mean time) image. Figure 2 shows the parenchymal factor time-activity curve after deconvolution and the pelvic factor time-activity curve.

Transit time measurements are shown in figure 3. Using the cortical ROI, half the hydronephrotic (but unobstructed) kidneys had markedly prolonged MPTT, presumably due to cross-talk from the dilated pelvis. With the cortical ROI, the deconvoluted curve often failed to return to baseline by the end of measurement (20 frames, 6.7 min) so that only a lower limit for the transit time could be calculated and plotted (open circles). When factor analysis rather than ROI was used to separate pelvic from parenchymal activity, the difference between normal and unobstructed hydronephrotic kidneys was much less (fig. 3). A small difference remained, suggesting that separation was still imperfect. When obstructed kidneys were compared with unobstructed hydronephrotic kidneys, three of the four obstructed kidneys had longer transit times than any unobstructed kidney (fig. 3), but the difference in this small series was not statistically significant.

The high court rates obtainable with ^{99m}Tc-MAG$_3$ readily permit operator-independent separation of cortical and pelvic activity by factor analysis, which appears preferable to manual ROI selection. The difference in parenchymal transit time between normal and chronically obstructed kidneys does not appear large enough to permit easy differentiation, but these preliminary data suggest that a larger series may reveal a statistically significant separation.

References

1 Verboven M, Achten R, Keuppens F, et al: Radioisotopic transit parameters in obstruction of pelviureteral junction. Urology 1989;32:370–374.
2 Barber DC: The use of principal components in the quantitative analysis of gamma camera dynamic studies. Phys Med Biol 1980;25:283–292.
3 Russell CD: Estimation of glomerular filtration rate using ^{99m}Tc-DTPA and the gamma camera. Eur J Nucl Med 1987;12:547–552.

C.D. Russell, MD, PhD, Division of Nuclear Medicine,
University of Alabama Hospital, 619 Nineteenth Street South,
Birmingham, AL 35233 (USA)

Blaufox MD, Hollenberg NK, Raynaud C (eds): Radionuclides in Nephro-Urology.
Contrib Nephrol. Basel, Karger, 1990, vol 79, pp 72–73

Renal Function Studies Using ^{99m}Tc-MAG$_3$: Pharmacokinetics and Slope Clearance Determination

B. Bubeck[a], *W. Brandau*[b], *E. Weber*[c], *S. Pomer*[d], *P. Georgi*[a], *K. zum Winkel*[a]

Departments of [a]Nuclear Medicine and [d]Urology, University of Heidelberg;
[b]Department of Nuclear Medicine, University of Münster, and
[c]Biostatistics, German Cancer Research Center, Heidelberg, FRG

The replacement of radioiodinated hippuric acid (OIH) by ^{99m}Tc-MAG$_3$ in renal function studies is generally expected and has, partially, already taken place. The major difference between both radiopharmaceuticals is the 1.5–fold higher plasma concentration of the Tc compound which is caused by its significantly higher protein binding as compared with OIH (approx. 90 vs. 70%). Considering the nearly identical elimination half-lives of both substances [1, 2], the clearance of Tc-MAG$_3$ is lower than that of OIH by a factor of 1.5 (simultaneous steady-state clearance measurement; n = 124). Because only the non-protein-bound fraction is ultrafiltered, only 2% of Tc-MAG$_3$ are eliminated by glomerular filtration. Therefore, the renal clearance of this substance is nearly equivalent to its 'tubular extraction rate' (TER) [2].

The amount of protein binding might be the reason for the different clearances: for Tc-MAG$_3$ the peritubular transit time is too short to dissociate this compound from the protein in percentages comparable with OIH. Therefore, the available portion of tubular extractable Tc-MAG$_3$ per renal passage is lower than that of OIH.

Under treatment with *p*-aminohippuric acid (PAH) the TER(MAG$_3$) is reduced by competitive inhibition to a significantly higher degree than the clearance of OIH. This can be an indication for a lower affinity of Tc-MAG$_3$ to the tubular transport system than the affinity of OIH. Nevertheless, no loss of information could be observed in transplant patients during periods of severely reduced renal function [3].

The plasma extraction efficiencies of both radiopharmaceuticals were determined simultaneously by the sampling of arterial and venous renal blood during unilateral nephrectomy in patients (n = 5). The comparison of these results with the preoperatively determined whole body clearances revealed that Tc-MAG_3 (HPLC-purified) is eliminated extrarenally just as little as OIH.

For determination of the TER(MAG_3) during slope, plasma concentrations were measured at different times within 45 min after single shot application (32 patients). Analogous to the Tauxe method [4], these concentrations were correlated to steady-state clearance data as reference, determined immediately afterwards (feedback-controlled infusion-pump system). It was shown that the standard deviations are within an acceptable range if the blood samples were taken not before the 20th min p.i. The following logarithmic function was found e.g. for blood drawn 25 min p.i.:

$$\text{TER}(\text{MAG}_3) = -509 + 229 \times \ln(\text{ID}/c_{25}) \quad [\text{ml/min}]$$

where ID = injected dose in MBq; c_{25} = plasma concentration 25 min p.i. in kBq/ml. The activity (kBq) of the plasma sample is calculated from the count rate using the calibration factor of the employed devices (relation well-type counter-to-dose calibrator).

With the calculated algorithms, it is possible to estimate the TER(MAG_3) by a single blood drawing and the accuracy is sufficient for clinical routine in the area above 50 ml/min. Taking into consideration the individual body dimensions, a further reduction of the standard deviation can be obtained (new algorithms are being developed). In comparison with camera-clearance measurements, this method has the advantage that it does not require a function study with a gamma camera, which constitutes a further source of error. But as all clearance measurements in slope, this method also represents a compromise between accuracy and practicability.

References

1 Taylor, AD Jr, Eshima AR, Fritzberg PE, et al: Comparison of iodine-131 OIH and technetium-99m-MAG_3, renal imaging in volunteers. J Nucl Med 1986;27:795–803.

2 Bubeck B, Brandau W, Eisenhut M, et al: The tubular extraction rate (TER) of Tc-99m-MAG_3: A new quatitative parameter of renal function. Nuc Compact 1987;18:260–267.

3 Bubeck B, Brandau W, Steinbächer M, et al: Technetium-99m-labeled renal function and imaging agents. II. Clinical evaluation of Tc-99m-MAG_3 (Tc-99m-mercaptoacetylglycylglycylglycine). Int J Radiat Appl Instrum – Nucl Med Biol 1988;15:109–118.

4 Tauxe WN, Dubovsky EV, Kidd T Jr, et al: New formulas for the calculation of effective renal plasma flow. Eur J Nucl Med 1982;7:51–54.

Bernd Bubeck, MD, BSc, Department of Nuclear Medicine, University of Heidelberg, Im Neuenheimer Feld 400, D–6900 Heidelberg (FRG)

Blaufox MD, Hollenberg NK, Raynaud C (eds): Radionuclides in Nephro-Urology.
Contrib Nephrol. Basel, Karger, 1990, vol 79, pp 74–76

The Impact of Different Urinary Flow Rates on Renoscintigraphy

J. Frøkiær, L. Knudsen, J. Mortensen, J.C. Djurhuus, F.T. Jensen
Institute of Experimental Clinical Research, University of Aarhus, and
Department of Clinical Physiology and Nuclear Medicine, Aarhus Municipal Hospital, Aarhus, Denmark

Deconvolution analysis of the renoscintigraphical data makes it possible to obtain the individual response from the kidney as the renal impulse retention function or mean transit time. This has important implication in a number of situations where renal function is impaired. However, interpretation of renal transit time is based on the assumption that the urine flow from both kidneys is the same and that no significant change in transit time occurs with changes in urine flow. However, parenchymal and pelvic transit times may vary considerably with diuresis. Previously it has been reported that there exists a hyperbolic relation between transit time and urine flow [1].

The aim of this study was therefore to investigate the influence of different urinary flow rates from each kidney on the parenchymal and pelvic transit time.

Material and Methods

Twenty pigs of Danish landrace were renoscintigraphied once a week for 4 weeks. The pigs were anesthetized with light halothane anesthesia (1.0–1.5%) induced by ketalar and midazolam i.m. The pigs were kept anesthetized in a semiclosed system with oxygen in 50% N_2O. Before renoscintigraphy, a cystoscope was placed in the bladder of the pig. The ureteral orifices were localized and a 5-F indwelling ureteral catheter was placed in each ureter with side and end holes placed in the pelvis of each kidney. To ensure that no leakage of urine took place, an indwelling urethral catheter was also placed in the bladder. Renoscintigraphy was done on a Siemens ZLC 7500 gamma camera and data collected in an on-line Nodecrest computer. The dose was 25 MBQ of ^{123}I-hippuran administrated i.v. and data collected in a 64 × 64 matrix, 80 frames of 20 s. The ROIs over each kidney were defined and the time activity curves and the background curve generated. Mean transit times were calculated from the impulse residual response using deconvolution for 15 min on the background-subtracted renograms.

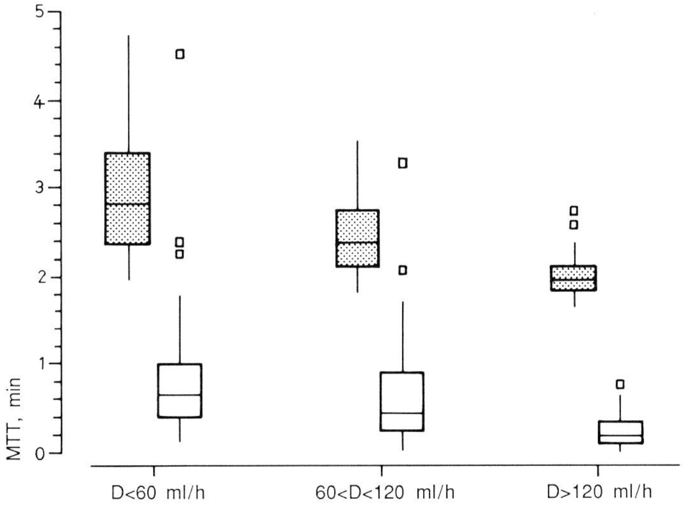

Fig. 1. Shown is a box-and-whiskers plot of the mean transit time (MTT) for the parenchyma (hatched bars) and the pelvis (open bars) in the three groups. Total range is shown, together with framed areas with median value and first quartile on each side. Extreme values exceeding 1.5 times interquartile length are plotted as individual points.

The pigs were hydrated in three different categories, so we obtained: (1) a group with oliguria by way of fluid deprivation 8 h prior to scintigraphy; (2) in normohydration the pigs had free access to water and were given 200 cm^3 i.v. prior and during the scintigraphy; (3) polyuria was obtained by giving the pigs free access to water and 500 cm^3 of saline i.v. prior to and during scintigraphy. Accordingly, we divided the animals or more precisely the kidneys and urinary tract systems into three different urinary flow intervals. Low flow: $D < 60$ ml/min, medium flow: $60 < D < 120$ ml/min, and high flow: $D > 120$ ml/min.

Statistical analysis: Data were analyzed by Student's t test and by one-way analysis of variance.

Results

All pigs had normal urinary tracts judged from the pictures from the gamma camera. The body weight of the animals averaged 30 kg at the start of the study. Looking at the parenchymal transit times at the different urinary flow intervals (fig. 1) there was a statistically significant difference between the three groups, $F = 33.2$, $p < 0.001$. Looking on the pelvic transit times (fig. 1) there was a similar statistically significant difference in transit time between the three groups, $F = 9.31$, $p = 0.0002$. Looking at the overall raw data distribution of mean transit times we found a wide variation in both parenchymal and pelvic transit times, with the highest standard deviation in the low urinary flow interval. No linear relationship between the mentioned parameters was found.

Discussion

In order to obtain valid deconvolution analysis we used ^{123}I-hippuran for the renoscintigraphies. We investigated normal kidneys and urinary tract systems in order to see what impact the urine flow had on parenchymal and pelvic transit times. These parameters are frequently used in clinical diagnosis of urological and nephrological disorders. However, urine production under these circumstances is often disturbed and reduced and we very seldom know the urine flow rate from each individual kidney. It is assumed that urine flow rate is equal from both kidneys and that it does not change from study to study. The latter is easy to measure. However, the urinary flow rate from each kidney is very rarely known. By catheterization of both ureters we got the exact urinary flow rate from each kidney. From the mean transit time raw data we find a large variation especially in the low urinary flow interval. This is clearly demonstrated in figure 1, and a significant reduction takes place in both MTT and standard deviation with increasing flow rates. The best results from deconvolution analysis are obtained in the group with high urinary flow rate.

Reference

1 Britton KE, Maisey MN: Renal radionuclide studies; in Maisey MN, Britton KE, Gilday DL (eds): Clinical Nuclear Medicine. Philadelphia, Saunders 1985, pp 93–133.

J. Frøkiær, MD, Institute of Experimental Clinical Research, University of Aarhus, Aarhus Municipal Hospital, DK-8000 Aarhus (Denmark)

Blaufox MD, Hollenberg NK, Raynaud C (eds): Radionuclides in Nephro-Urology.
Contrib Nephrol. Basel, Karger, 1990, vol 79, pp 77–81

Renal Function, Urinary Flow Rates and Diuresis Renography

S.C.W. Brown, S.M. Upsdell, C.D. Betts, P.H. O'Reilly
Department of Urology, Stepping Hill Hospital, Stockport, Cheshire, UK

Over the past 10 years, diuresis renography has become an established method for the investigation of upper tract dilatation when obstruction is suspected [1]. During renography, a dilated system may be confirmed as obstructive or nonobstructive dilatation by the administration of a diuretic (furosemide) 20 min after the radiopharmaceutical – standard (F + 20) diuresis renography. In a proportion of cases, the result remains equivocal. Further clarification of these can be obtained in many cases by employing the modification of injecting the diuretic 15 min before the radiopharmaceutical, the F – 15 method [2].

Two factors may contribute to poor wash-out after frusemide during diuresis renography. If renal function is very low, there may be reduced uptake of the tracer, and the kidney may be unable to respond to the diuretic with an adequate flow rate. If the collecting system volume is massive, wash-out may be sluggish due to mixing chamber effects [3]. Both these factors may also contribute to reported discrepancies between diuresis renography and perfusion pressure flow studies.

This paper examines the relationship between renal function and the urinary flow rate induced by furosemide to assess whether knowledge of renal function can assist in the interpretation of the diuresis renogram. Emphasis has been placed on the urinary flow rate 3–6 and 15–18 min after the diuretic injection. The 3- to 6-min interval is of relevance to standard diuresis renography when the early effect of the diuretic on the rising curve is under study. The 15- to 18-min period relates to renography when the furosemide is given 15 min before the radiopharmaceutical to achieve maximum diuresis.

Table 1. Product moment correlation coefficients for the relationships between the three parameters of renal function and the urinary flow rates for the two time periods; also given are the predicted clearance values with 95% confidence limits which would be expected to correspond to a total urinary flow rate of 20 ml/min

Clearance	Urinary flow rates			
	3- to 6-min period		15- to 18-min period	
	correlation coefficient	predicted clearance for 20 ml/min flow	correlation coefficient	predicted clearance for 20 ml/min flow
Creatinine clearance	0.66***	77 ± 45	0.775***	68 ± 38
Tc-DTPA clearance	0.66***	56 ± 24	0.77***	51 ± 21
^{123}I-hippuran clearance	0.59**	298 ± 183	0.71***	269 ± 158

*** = $p < 0.001$; ** = $p < 0.01$.

Patients and Methods

84 male and 2 female patients were studied. All had indwelling urethral catheters either prior to, or after elective urological procedures. All were normally hydrated and in a stable medical condition. 15 min before the study, each patient was given 500 ml of water to drink. The patients were then placed supine, the catheter bags disconnected, the bladder allowed to empty and a steady flow rate established. The minute-by-minute flow rate was then measured over 30 min using graduated measuring cylinders. 40 mg of furosemide was injected intravenously after the second minute.

39 patients had creatinine clearances performed, 27 had a more accurate measure of glomerular filtration rate (GFR) and in 20, effective renal plasma flow was measured. In all but 2 cases, these clearance studies were performed the same day as the flow rate measurement. The 24-hour urine sample for creatinine clearance was collected through the catheter and timed to end just before the start of the flow rate analysis when the plasma sample was taken. GFR was measured as the plasma clearance of ^{99m}Tc-diethylene triamine penta-acetic acid (Tc-DTPA), using a two-sample, single-injection method following routine protocol adopted in this department. To measure effective renal plasma flow, the single sample, V_{44} method for ^{123}iodo-hippuran clearance was performed at the same time as standard renography [4].

Results

The average urinary flow rate at 3–6 min was 20.5 ml/min and at 15–18 min was 24.0 ml/min. This difference was highly significant ($p < 0.001$). Table 1 gives the Pearson product moment correlation coefficients for the relationships between the creatinine, ^{99m}Tc-DTPA and ^{123}-iodo-hippuran clearances, and the flow rates at 3–6 and 15–18 min.

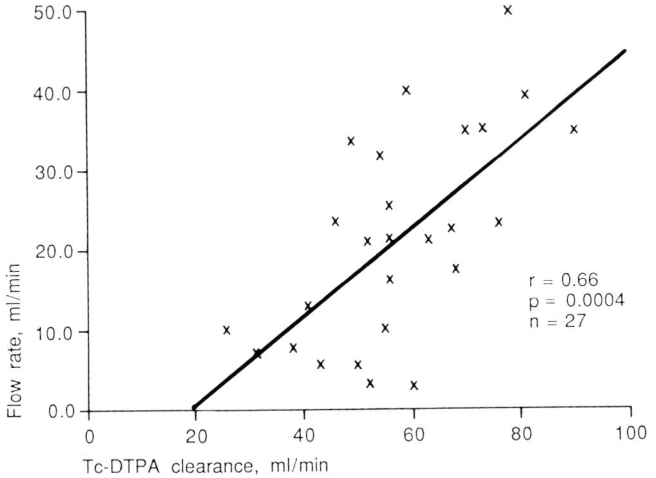

1

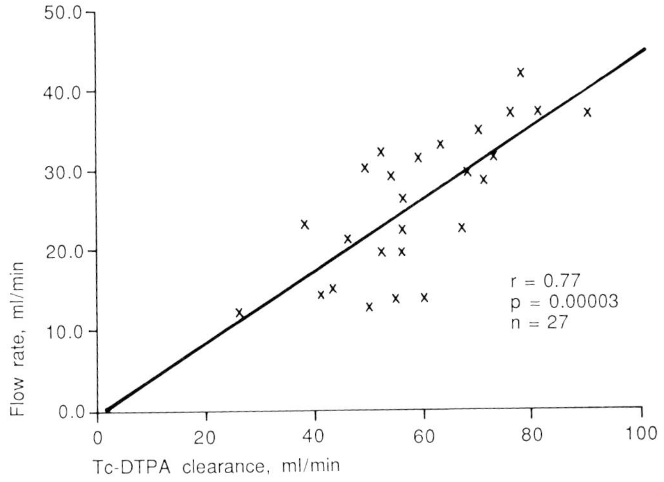

2

Fig. 1. Scattergraph with line of best fit for the relationship between Tc-DTPA clearance and the total urinary flow rate for the 3- to 6-min period.

Fig. 2. Scattergraph with line of best fit for the relationship between Tc-DTPA clearance and the total urinary flow rate for the 15- to 18-min period.

Figures 1 and 2 are scattergraphs of Tc-DTPA clearance versus the flow during the 3- to 6-min period and the 15- to 18-min period respectively. As with the other parameters of renal function, the scatter is considerable particularly at the 3- to 6-min interval. The correlations are however highly significant for all studies.

Discussion

Diuresis renography and perfusion pressure flow studies are the two main methods used for the assessment of dilatation of the upper urinary tract. Diuresis renography will give an unequivocal result in approximately 85% of cases, but disagreement has been reported between the two techniques. In recent series, agreement has varied between 53% [5] and 85% [6]. There is both underestimation and overestimation of obstruction relative to both techniques. A number of these discrepancies may be due to differences in the flow rates achieved during the two tests.

Regression analyses applied to our figures (table 1) indicate that, at 3–6 min, to ensure a total flow of 20 ml/min, i.e. a single kidney flow rate of 10 ml/min as used in perfusion pressure flow studies, the patient's creatinine clearance should be in the order of 77 ml/min and Tc-DTPA clearance to be in the order of 56 ml/min. At a clearance of 32 ml/min for both types of GFR measurement, there would be only a 1 in 20 chance of achieving this. 15–18 min after frusemide, the corresponding clearance values are less, though because of the tighter distribution, there is little difference in the lower 95% confidence limits. The higher values for the creatinine compared with the DTPA and contrast clearance reflect the tendency for creatinine clearance to overestimate the GFR, particularly at lower levels.

These results would suggest that the results of diuresis renography in patients with a total GFR of less than 30 ml/min should be examined critically. They may give an unequivocal result for clinical guidance but without necessarily agreeing with perfusion pressure flow studies because of the differences in urinary flow rates. Attention to the physiological principles underlying the available tests for the assessment of urinary tract dilatation is necessary to achieve the most reliable interpretation of their results.

References

1 O'Reilly PH, Lawson RS, Shields RA, et al: Idiopathic hydronephrosis – the diuresis renogram: a new non-invasive method of assessing equivocal pelviureteric junction obstruction. J Urol 1979;121:153.

2 English PH, Testa HJ, Shields RA, et al: Modified method of diuresis renography for the assessment of equivocal pelviureteric junction obstruction. Br J Urol 1987;59:10–14.

3 Kletter K, Nurnburger N: Diagnostic potential of diuresis renography: limitations by the severity of hydronephrosis and impairment of renal function. Nucl Med Commun 1989;10:51–61.

4 O'Reilly PH, Shields RA, Testa HJ: Radiopharmaceuticals in Nuclear Medicine in Urology and Nephrology, ed 2. London, Butterworth, 1981, pp 49–59.
5 Whitaker RH, Buxton-Thomas MS: A comparison of pressure flow studies and renography in equivocal upper urinary tract obstruction. J Urol 1984;131:446.
6 Kass EJ, Majd M, Belman AB: Comparison of the diuretic renogram and the pressure perfusion study in children. J Urol 1985;134:92.

P.H. O'Reilly, Department of Urology, Stepping Hill Hospital,
Stockport, Cheshire SK2 7JE (UK)

Blaufox MD, Hollenberg NK, Raynaud C (eds): Radionuclides in Nephro-Urology.
Contrib Nephrol. Basel, Karger, 1990, vol 79, pp 82–86

Validation of a New Method for Quantifying Renal Function

G. La Cava, R. Sciagrà, A.R. Formiconi, U. Meldolesi

Department of Clinical Pathophysiology, Nuclear Medicine,
University of Florence, Italy

Several methods have been proposed for the calculation of the effective renal plasma flow (ERPF) and glomerular filtration rate (GFR) using the clearance of radiolabelled tracers during renal sequential scintigraphy (RSS) [1]. Methods based on external measurements only (gamma camera methods) appear particularly attractive because they are simple and rapid. They are, however, subject to many possible sources of error, which need to be considered, and their validation with an accurate reference method is mandatory [2]. In a previous report we described our approach, which was validated with good results with a reliable clearance calculation method [3]. In this study we evaluated a further refinement of the background subtraction technique and the introduction of correction factors for the influences produced by kidney depth and surface dimensions on the system counting efficiency.

Methods

RSS was perfomed with the patient supine, using a large field of view gamma camera (ZLC, Siemens) equipped with a medium energy (360 KeV) collimator and interfaced with a Hewlett-Packard A900 computer. The syringe with the dose to be injected (222 kBq/kg body weight of ^{131}I-hippuran) was previously counted with the gamma camera after being positioned on a special 6-cm thick plexiglas support placed on the examination bed. After injection, a 28-min study was acquired in list mode with a 5-s resolution and subsequently rearranged in 5-s frames on a 64×64 matrix. A precordial time/activity curve was simultaneously registered using a computer interfaced single probe placed over the precordium.

According to our previously published report [3], the single kidney ^{131}I-hippuran clearance is related to the fraction of tracer accumulated by the kidney during the first minute after administration (D_1), which can be calculated by dividing the radioactivity measured in each renal region of interest (ROI) by the injected dose.

The renal ROIs were extracted using an automated threshold algorithm. The background was subtracted taking into account the intravascular radioactivity, which is significant in the first 2 min after injection according to the formula:

$$R(t) = g\,P(t) + h \int_o^t P(t)\,dt$$

where R(t) is the renal time/activity curve, P(t) is the precordial curve, g a constant determined with the least square method, h the coefficient used to normalize the precordial curve to the renal tracing, and where gP(t) represents the background contribution to the renal curve in the first minutes. The deformation of the radioactive bolus during the transit from the heart to the kidney was taken into account and to this aim the precordial time/activity curve was convoluted with a random walk function [W(t)] [4]. After subtracting of the gP(t)·W(t), the D_l of the single kidney is expressed by the formula:

$$D_l = \frac{h \int_o^t P(t) \cdot W(t) d}{S}$$

where S is the injected dose measured by counting the preinjection syringe.

The influence of kidney surface dimensions and depth on the system counting efficiency was determined using phantoms (^{131}I sources of different diameter positioned at increasing depth in a tissue-like attenuation medium) and the appropriate correction factors were calculated and introduced in the computer program. In the processing of the single patient study the kidney surface dimensions were evaluated from the number of pixels included in the renal ROIs. The kidney depth was estimated using a lateral scintigram: the distance in pixel between the middle of the renal image and a linear source positioned on the examination bed was measured and multiplied by the pixel length (6 mm). Then the related data are employed in the correction formula as follows:

$$E(d, s) = e^{(-0.14d)} s^{(0.06 + 0.0057d)}$$

where E = system efficiency, d = kidney depth in cm, s = kidney area in pixel (fig. 1).

Finally an appropriate correction factor for the attenuation by the soft tissues of the employed radionuclide photons was included in the computer program in order to allow its use indifferently with ^{99m}Tc, ^{131}I or ^{123}I.

The study group for the validation of our method included 25 patients (19 males and 6 females, age range 17–74), affected by various nephrourologic problems and addressed to our laboratory for the evaluation of renal function. All of them underwent renal sequential scintigraphy according to the above described procedure. In 20 subjects the renal sequential scintigraphy was repeated using ^{123}I-hippuran (74 MBq) after a short time interval, without intervening changes in clinical conditions and in the blood parameters monitoring renal function; the comparison of the two evaluations was used to estimate the reproducibility of our technique.

For calculation of the clearance according to Sapirstein et al. [5], blood was withdrawn through a teflon indwelling cannula inserted in an antecubital vein at 2, 4, 6, 8, 10, 17, 24, 34, 44 and 54 min after injection of the tracer. One-milliliter plasma samples were counted in a well-counter, the results were plotted on semilogarithmic paper to identify the two exponential components of the concentration curve and the clearance was calculated according to the usual formula [5].

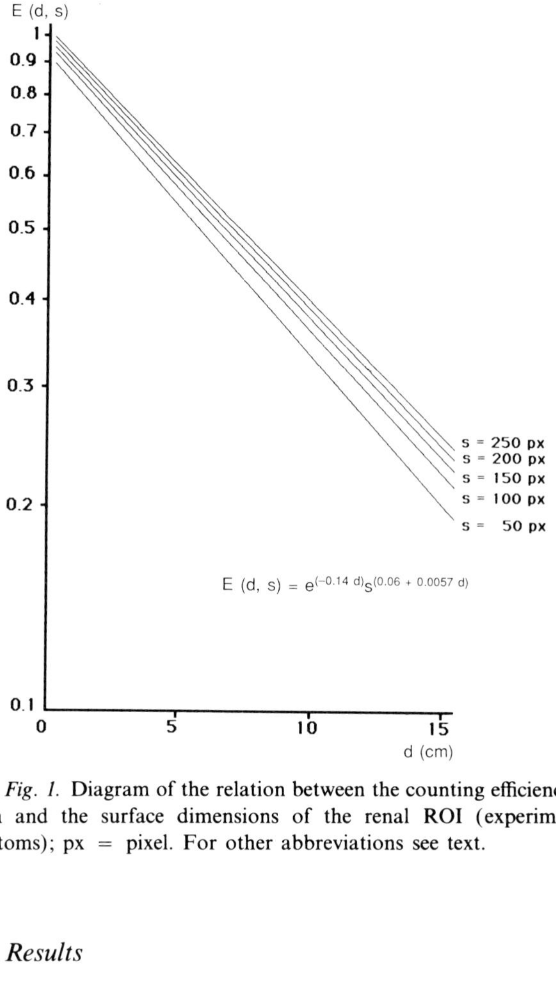

Fig. 1. Diagram of the relation between the counting efficiency of the system, the kidney depth and the surface dimensions of the renal ROI (experimental data obtained using phantoms); px = pixel. For other abbreviations see text.

Results

The linear regression analysis of the comparison between the ^{131}I-hippuran clearance calculated according to Sapirstein et al. [5], and the sum of the single kidney D_1 of each patient (D_1s) subtracted of background and corrected for depth and surface dimensions yielded the following results: Clearance (Sapirstein) = 10 + 3182 D_1s, $r = 0.97$ ($p < 0.00001$) (fig. 2). Therefore a close correlation between the two values could be demonstrated and a proportionality factor was established (i.e. 3182), which transforms the D_1 in the related ^{131}I-hippuran clearance and therefore allows the calculation of the single kidney ERPF on the basis of external measurements only. The same correction factor allows the calculation of the ERPF

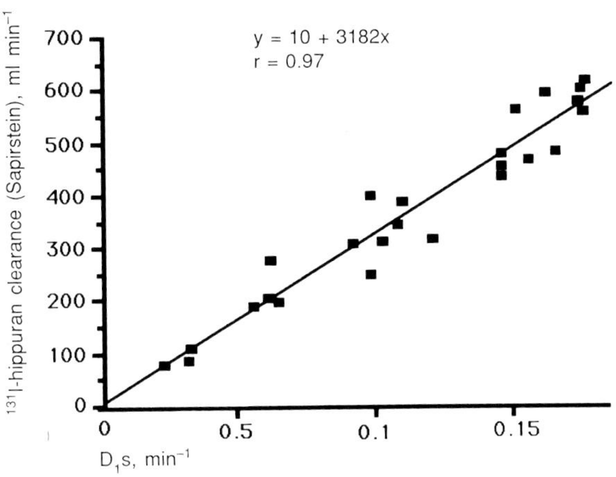

Fig. 2. Comparison of the sum of the two single kidney D_1 (D_1s) and the ^{131}I-hippuran clearance measured according to Sapirstein et al. [5].

also using ^{123}I-hippuran. With regard to reproducibility of our method, the comparison of the paired evaluations in 20 cases showed the following linear regression analysis result: ^{123}I-hippuran $D_1 = 19 + 0.91$ ^{131}I-hippuran D_1, $r = 0.94$ ($p < 0.00001$).

Discussion

Gamma camera methods for the quantification of renal function offer the advantage of ease and rapidity. On the other hand, they are subject to the influence of various sources of error [1] and therefore are usually classified as less accurate when compared with the procedures based on blood samples counting [2]. In our approach, however, we tried to take into account some of the more relevant causes of inaccuracy of the gamma camera methods. Among them there is certainly the background subtraction: methods using background ROIs give substantially different results depending on the location of the ROI [2]. Our background subtraction technique overcomes this problem, without apparently affecting the accuracy of the data. The influence of kidney depth and surface dimensions on the system counting efficiency is another crucial point for quantitative measurements [1, 2]. In our approach both variables were measured in the individual patient and the appropriate correction factors automatically selected by the computer processing among those previously determined with phantom studies. Since our method is based on the kidney tracer uptake during the first minute, the influences due to renal function and type of employed radiopharmaceutical should be negligible. Theoretically it is therefore possible to use it also with glomerular filtration tracers. As a matter of fact, preliminary data with ^{99m}Tc-DTPA correlated well with the ERPF calculation, with a proportionality factor of 0.19, the same value of filtration fraction in humans.

As a final remark, the good results of the direct comparison between our procedure and an accurate gold standard need to be stressed, because this is the necessary confirmation of the value of every method proposed for quantifying renal function.

References

1 Dubovsky EV, Russell CD: Quantitation of renal function with glomerular and tubular agents. Semin Nucl Med 1982;12:308–329.

2 Fine EJ, Axelrod M, Gorkin J, et al: Measurement of effective renal plasma flow: a comparison of methods. J Nucl Med 1987;28:1393–1400.

3 Formiconi AR, La Cava G, Morotti A, et al: Renal sequential scintigraphy: unilateral clearance rate determination based on external measurements only. Eur J Nucl Med 1983;8:150–154.

4 Sheppard CW: Basic Principles of the Tracer Method Introduction to the Mathematical Tracer Kinetics. New York, Wiley, 1962.

5 Sapirstein LA, Vidt DG, Mandel MJ, et al: Volumes of distribution and clearances of intravenously injected creatinine in the dog. Am J Physiol 1955;180:330–336.

Giuseppe La Cava, MD, Department of Clinical Pathophysiology, Nuclear Medicine, University of Florence, Viale Morgagni 85, I–50134 Florence (Italy)

Blaufox MD, Hollenberg NK, Raynaud C (eds): Radionuclides in Nephro-Urology.
Contrib Nephrol. Basel, Karger, 1990, vol 79, pp 87–98

The Radionuclide Renal Scan: Past, Present and Future[1]

Leonard M. Freeman
Montefiore Medical Center and Albert Einstein College of Medicine, Bronx, N.Y., USA

The development of the scintillation scanner in 1950 [1] heralded the birth of the modern era of radionuclide imaging. According to Winter [1], Goodwin was the first to attempt a renal scan with the use of ^{131}I-labeled diodrast. A similar attempt was made by Winter, himself, in 1955. In both instances, the rapid excretion of the diodrast did not allow for the 30 or more minutes needed to scan the kidneys with the small detector system available. Winter did meet with success in rabbit studies following ureteral ligation.

In the late 1950s, considerable interest was generated in a new study performed with individual scintillation probes over each kidney that monitored the transit of radioiodinated orthoiodohippurate through each kidney – the renogram [2, 3]. At the University of Michigan, Haynie et al. [4] used constant infusions of hippuran to image experimentally-produced renal infarcts in dogs. In 1963, Schlegel et al. [5] at Tulane artificially created 'stop flow' conditions with occluding bilateral ureteral catheters. This kept the hippuran in the kidneys long enough to perform the rectilinear imaging study (fig. 1). Physiologic alterations such as obstructive uropathy and azotemia also provided prolonged renal transit of the radiohippuran. This allowed several investigators such as Wenzl et al. [6], Rosenthall [7] and Freeman et al, [8] to obtain successful static imaging studies.

The first radiopharmaceutical that actually bound in the kidney was ^{203}Hg-chlormerodrin developed by Borghraef and Pitts [9] in 1956. High concentration of this agent was identified in the renal cortex of animals

[1] Special invited paper.

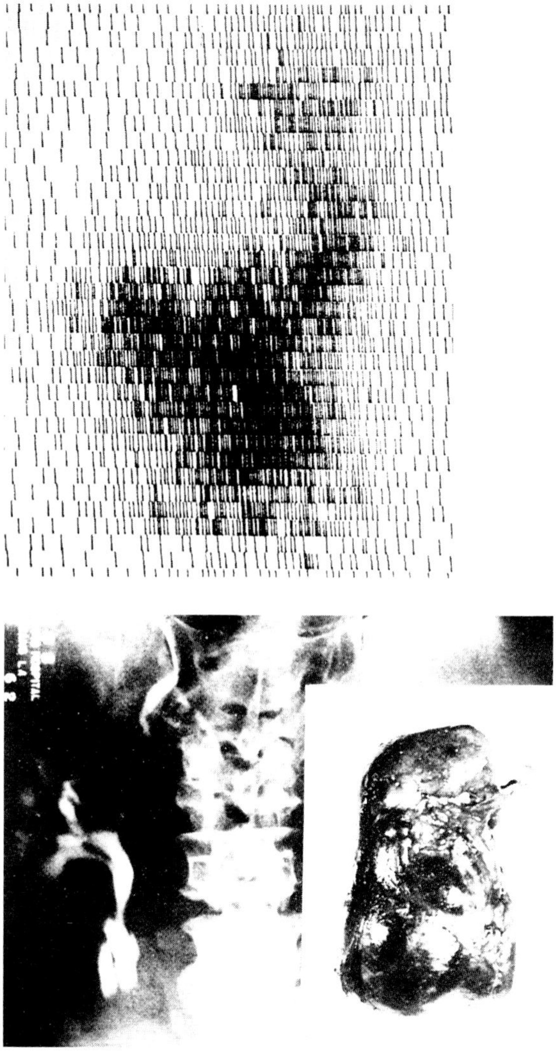

a

b

Fig. 1. 'Stop flow' technique for radiohippuran rectilinear scanning. Following right retrograde catheterization and ureteral blockage, a good radiohippuran image is obtained. *a* Absent uptake is seen in the upper pole of the right kidney. *b* Radiographic and pathologic specimens confirm the presence of a cyst [from 5, with permission].

1–2 h following intravenous administration. Interestingly, the first human application of ^{203}Hg-chlormerodrin was in brain scanning by Blau and Bender [10] in 1959. McAfee and Wagner [11] quickly followed with the first kidney scans using this agent in 1960. At this point, many clinical applications were conceived and use became widespread. Because of its dosimetric advantages, ^{197}Hg-chlormerodrin introduced by Sodee [12] in 1963 became that era's agent of choice for renal scanning.

In the mid and late 1960s, the introduction of technetium-99m chemistry into clinical nuclear medicine insured the success of Anger's scintillation camera as the modern-day standard in nuclear medicine instrumentation. Technetium's 140 KeV monochromatic gamma emission and short 6-hour physical half-life was a perfect partner for the larger and thinner NaI crystal of the Anger camera. For the first time, compact bolus injections of higher amounts of activity allowed for rapid multi-second image exposures and the visualization of vascular pathways throughout the body – the radionuclide angiogram. Rosenthall [13] and Powell and Anger [14] were the first to apply this technique to kidney imaging.

Quantitative determination of individual renal function was a by-product of renal scintigraphy, particularly with those agents that became fixed in the renal parenchyma for long periods of time. Although it is not the purpose of this author to review such quantitative methods, one particular piece of elegant work deserves historic mention since it involved an imaging agent primarily used in Europe. This was Raynaud and coworkers [15] use of ^{197}Hg-bichloride for measuring the functional integrity of each kidney. This study initially was performed with external probes and subsequently was successfully converted to rectilinear scan and Anger camera methodology. It was the forerunner of similar studies currently performed with the various ^{99m}Tc renal agents.

In the 1970s, several ^{99m}Tc-labeled compounds were developed (table 1). Three of these proved useful. These were glucoheptonate (GHA), 2,3-dimercaptosuccinic acid (DMSA) and dimethylenetriamine pentaacetic acid (DTPA). Arnold et al. [16] have thoroughly reviewed the biokinetics of these three agents. In brief, DTPA primarily is excreted through the glomerular filtrate while GHA and DMSA bind to the renal tubules in varying degrees. The reader is referred to the excellent article by Arnold et al. [16] which thoroughly reviews and compares the biokinetics of these three agents.

In the early 1980s, several diamide disulfur (DADS) ligands for ^{99m}Tc were developed and evaluated [17]. They proved to be inferior to hippuran in terms of specificity and excretory rate in both normal and azotemic patients. The most significant recent development in renal radio-

Table 1. Selected historical aspects of renal scintigraphy

1	^{131}I-diodrast [Goodwin and Winter, 1955]
2	^{131}I-hippuran A Normals Constant infusion [Haynie 1961] 'Stop flow' [Izenstark and Schlegel, 1962] B Abnormals Obstructive uropathy [Wenzl, 1963] Azotemia [Rosenthall, 1966; Powell and Anger, 1966]
3	^{203}Hg-chlormerodrin Developed by Borghgraef and Phipps [1956] Initially used as brain agent [Blau and Bender 1959] First renal images [McAfee and Wagner, 1960]
4	^{197}Hg-chlormerodrin Introduced by Sodee [1963] Anger camera images [Gottschalk 1965]
5	^{99m}Tc-pertechnetate perfusion scans [Rosenthall et al., 1966].
6	^{99m}Tc-gluconate [Charamza and Budikova, 1969] ^{99m}Tc-glucoheptonate [New Engl Nucl Rev 1974–6]
7	^{99m}Tc-Fe ascorbic acid complex [Winston et al., 1971]
8	^{99m}Tc-DTPA [Hauser et al., 1970]
9	^{99m}Tc-penicillamine-acetazolamide complex [Halpern et al., 1972]
10	^{99m}Tc-dimercaptosuccinic acid (DMSA) [Englander et al., 1974]
11	^{99m}Tc-DADS [Davison and Jones, formulated in 1981; McAfee et al., used in 1984]
12	^{99m}Tc-mercaptoacetyltriglycine (MAG_3) [Fritzberg et al., 1986]

pharmaceuticals is ^{99m}Tc-mercaptoacetyltriglycine (MAG_3) which appears to be that long sought after ^{99m}Tc-labeled substitute for hippuran [18]. It is believed that FDA approval in the United States will be forthcoming sometime in 1990. The agent is in general use throughout the rest of the world. Table 1 summarizes some of the most significant historical developments in renal scintigraphy.

The Present

The current state-of-the-art scintigraphic examination allows us to examine three areas of kidney function. These are perfusion, functional morphology and excretion.

Perfusion

The use of a small volume, high activity bolus (approx. 10 mCi) of ^{99m}Tc-labeled agent and a scintillation camera allows visualization of the abdominal aorta and the kidneys during the first 30 s following injection. Most often, renal specific radiopharmaceuticals such as ^{99m}Tc-DTPA, GHA or MAG_3 are employed since follow-through images could then be used to evaluate morphology (GHA) or excretion (DTPA or MAG_3). The greater degree of fixation and associated higher radiation dose per administered mCi of ^{99m}Tc-DMSA contraindicate its use for such 'flow' studies. This latter agent has found its greatest use in assessing individual renal function and performing single photon emission computed tomography (SPECT) studies of the kidney [19].

Functional Morphology

The most common radiopharmaceutical used for static, fixation-type renal examinations is ^{99m}Tc-GHA. As mentioned above, ^{99m}Tc-DMSA also is frequently used (particularly in Europe) for these types of exams, especially when SPECT is performed [19]. Since the fixation per administered mCi of DMSA is 3–4 times greater than GHA, the dose of the former can be held at 2–3 mCi instead of the usual 10-mCi dose of GHA given for the perfusion study. This exam has been primarily utilized to elucidate questionable or equivocal radiologic findings, e.g. mass lesions and infarcts, and distinguish between true space-occupying lesions and anatomic variants, e.g. column of Bertini.

Excretion

Orthoidodohippurate labeled with ^{123}I and ^{99m}Tc-DTPA are the major radiopharmaceuticals used for evaluating excretory function. The former is preferred by this author because of its more rapid and predictable handling by both glomerular filtration and tubular secretion. Figure 2 is a typical study performed at the Montefiore Medical Center. Semiquantitative analysis of hippuran uptake during the first 3 min of the study allows a rough estimate of individual renal function. This is included in the upper right-hand portion of the figure and is a routine determination at our institution. As indicated above, it is anticipated that ^{99m}Tc-MAG_3 will progressively replace the use of radioiodinated hippuran over the next few years.

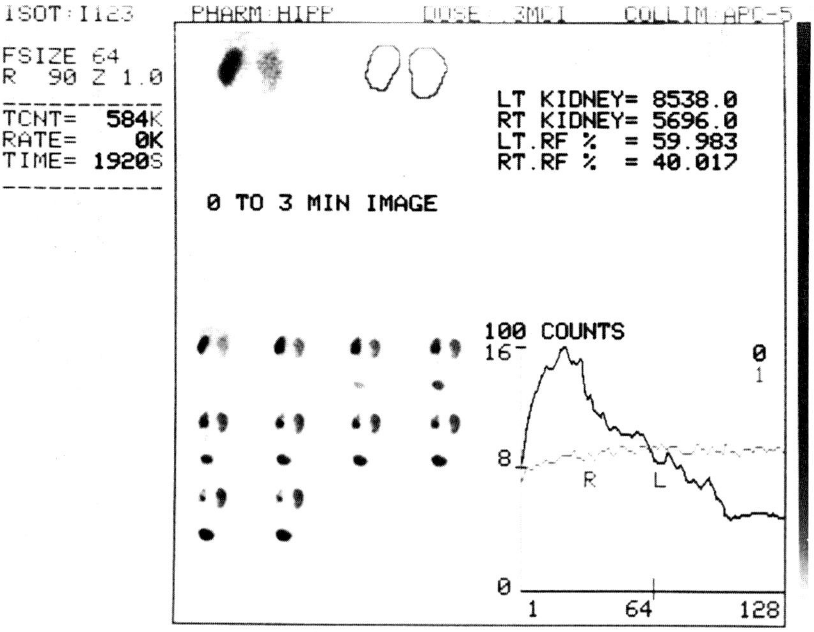

Fig. 2. Current ^{123}I-hippuran scintirenogram as performed at Montefiore Medical Center. The patient has a chronic right obstructive uropathy. Serial 3-min images show delayed uptake and excretion on right. The semiquantitative analysis of individual renal function displayed on the upper right is a routine part of every study.

Interventional Studies

Two pharmacologic interventions have had significant impact on improving the information yield from our routine radionuclide imaging studies of the kidney. These are furosemide diuretic studies (to distinguish functional dilatation from true anatomic obstruction) [20, 21] and captopril-enhanced studies (to enhance the detection of renovascular hypertension) [22, 23]. One physiologic intervention that has received some interest is Clorius' use of postural change and stress to demonstrate otherwise unsuspected unilateral and bilateral changes in renal transit [24, 25].

The Future

Three areas lend themselves to some discussion concerning what we might look for in the 1990s. These are SPECT, positron emission tomography (PET) and radioimmunoimaging.

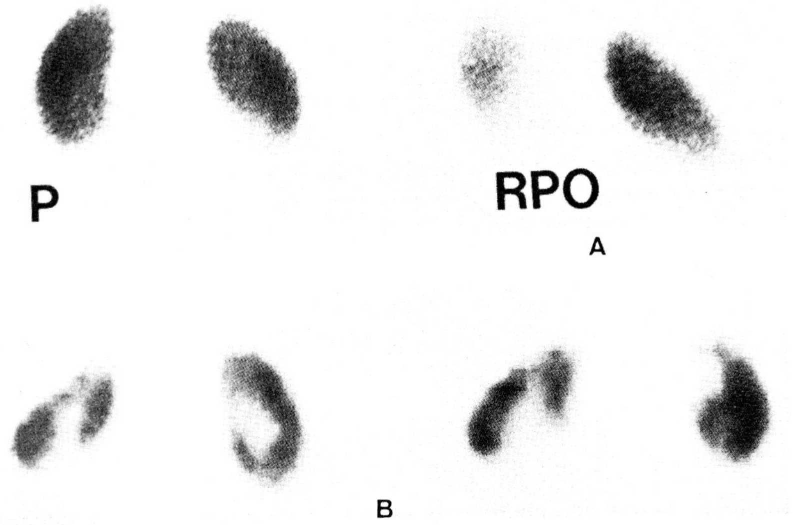

Fig. 3. Value of SPECT in elucidating renal space-occupying disease. Upper row: planar posterior and right posterior oblique images with ^{99m}Tc-DMSA show slightly reduced uptake in the lower pole of the right kidney; lower row: coronal tomographic sections show a more definitive defect [from 19, with permission].

Single Photon Tomography

As mentioned earlier, SPECT kidney imaging already has been performed in a few centers [19, 26]. The radiopharmaceutical most often used has been DMSA although GHA also is suitable. It major use thus far has been to determine whether the detection of space-occupying lesions can be enhanced. Williams et al. [19] compared planar and tomographic images from 60 patients suspected of having space-occupying lesions of the kidney. They found that there was not an overall statistically significant improvement in detection rate. However its use in specific selected circumstances such as obese patients, and those with equivocal urographic studies as well as its combination with a perfusion study considerably enhanced its value. This experience is still very preliminary and, undoubtedly, forthcoming reports will help determine SPECT's appropriate role in investigating various renal disorders. Figure 3 is an example of a renal cyst that is seen more clearly on tomographic rather than planar images.

Positron Emission Tomography

Quantification of arterial blood flow has been the primary area upon which initial renal PET investigations have focused. Following Yano and

Table 2. Monoclonal antibodies to kidney antigens

mAb (Ig class)	Defined antigen	Site of expression	Laboratory
T138 (IgM)	gp25[1]	vascular endothelium	MSKCC[2]
J143/URO-1 (IgG_1)	gp140, 120, 30	glomerulus, urothelium	MSKCC
AJ8 (IgG_1)	gp100 (CALLA[3])	glomerulus, proximal tubule (PT)	MSKCC
S4/URO-2 (IgG_{2a})	gp160	glomerulus, PT	MSKCC
T43/URO-10 (IgG_1)	gp85	PT	MSKCC
F23/URO-3 (IgG_{2a})	gp140	PT	MSKCC
S23/URO-4a (IgG_1)	gp120 (ADAbp[4])	PT, loop of Henle (LH)	MSKCC
S27/URO-4 (IgG_1)	gp120 (ADAbp)	PT, LH	MSKCC
S6 (IgG_1)	gp120 (ADAbp)	PT, LH	MSKCC
F31/URO-8 (IgM)	glycolipid	PT[5], LH	MSKCC
C26 (IgG_{2a})	gp40	distal tubule (DT), collecting tubule (CT), urothelium	MSKCC
M2 (IgM)	A-blood group	CT, urothelium	MSKCC
S8 (IgM)	B-blood group	CT, urothelium	MSKCC
T16 (IgG_{2b})	gp48, 42	DT, CT, urothelium	MSKCC
S22 (IgG_1)	gp115	renal cancer only	MSKCC
10.32 (IgG_1)	gp90 (TammHorsfall)	LH, DT	Cedarlane Labs
OKIal (IgG_2)	HLA-DR	endothelium, mesangium	Ortho Pharm.
Anti-SSEA-1 (IgM)	glycolipid	PT	Wistar Inst.
A6H (IgG_1)	ND	PT	U. Minn.
D5D (IgG_1)	ND	Bowman's capsule (BC)	U. Minn.
C5H (IgG_1)	p115	glomerulus	U. Minn.
Anti-B1 (IgG_{2a})	ND	fetal ureteral bud	Dana-Farber
BA-1 (IgM)	ND	BC, DT, CT,	U. Minn.
BA-2 (IgG_3)	p24	BC, DT, CT	U. Minn.
E6 (ND)	ND	renal cancer only	Mainz, FRG
B7 (ND)	ND	renal cancer only	Mainz, FRG
C8 (ND)	ND	renal cancer only	Mainz, FRG
D8 (ND)	ND	renal cancer only	Mainz, FRG
DU-ALL-1	p24	glomerulus[6], DT	Duke Univ.
DU-HL60-4	p160	PT, BC	Duke Univ.
DU-HL60-3 (IgM)	p15	PT[7]	Duke Univ.

ND = not defined.
[1] gp25 = glycoprotein; 25,000 molecular weight.
[2] MSKCC = Memorial Sloan-Kettering Cancer Center.
[3] CALLA = common acute lymphoblastic leukemia antigen.
[4] ADAbp = adenosine deaminase binding protein.
[5] Pars recta only.
[6] Mesangial cells.
[7] Pars recta convoluted.

Anger's [27] lead with 82 Rb and planar scintillation camera imaging, Tamaki et al. [28] used the same positron emitter and modern PET methodology. They demonstrated flow changes in a unilateral renal artery stenosis model before and after captopril administration [29]. Other efforts at studying blood flow to the kidney with PET have been initiated using tracers such as ^{11}C-albumin microspheres [30], $H_2{}^{15}O$ [31] and ^{62}Cu(II)-bis-(N^4-methylthiosemicarbazone) (CuPTSM) [32].

In studying metabolic function of the kidney, one must recognize the potential problem associated with normal uptake and excretion of the radiopharmaceutical being studied. This is typified by ^{18}FDG, which has been used to study tumor invasion with autoradiographic techniques. Fluorodeoxyglucose is handled by the kidney in a complex fashion that appears to involve filtration, tubular reabsorption and excretion in addition to its metabolic rate related processes. Other metabolic related renal studies have utilized ^{68}Ga-dehydroxyanthranquinones [34], phenolic amino carboxylic acid [35], a cluster ion complex of copper and penicillamine [36] and ^{68}Ga-EDTA [37].

The study of cellular growth and division in renal cell carcinoma has been looked at with ^{13}N-ammonia [38]. As with FDG studies, normal uptake and excretion of labeled amino acids, nucleic acids and their precursors often is very high and can be difficult to differentiate from a true metabolic uptake of the labeled compound.

It is clear that we are still in the very early stages of PET studies of the kidney although there definitely is enthusiasm for some of the ongoing investigations, particularly those dealing with the quantification of arterial blood flow.

Radioimmunoimaging

The use of labeled monoclonal antibodies in renal basic science research has not progressed as rapidly as it has in other organ and disease process areas of investigation. Bander [39] recently wrote an extensive review of exciting ongoing research involving antibodies and the kidney. He lists a total of 31 monoclonal antibodies to specific kidney antigens that have been described (fig. 4). Specific sites of expression in the nephron for each of these antibodies allows one to construct an antigenic map of the kidney (table 2). A particular cell can have its antigenic phenotype defined by determining whether these antigens are present or not [39]. Most of the work performed up until this time has focused primarily on developing monoclonal antibodies to renal cell carcinoma [40]. As in other areas of radiolabeled antibody investigations, success will carry important and exciting therapeutic potential as well.

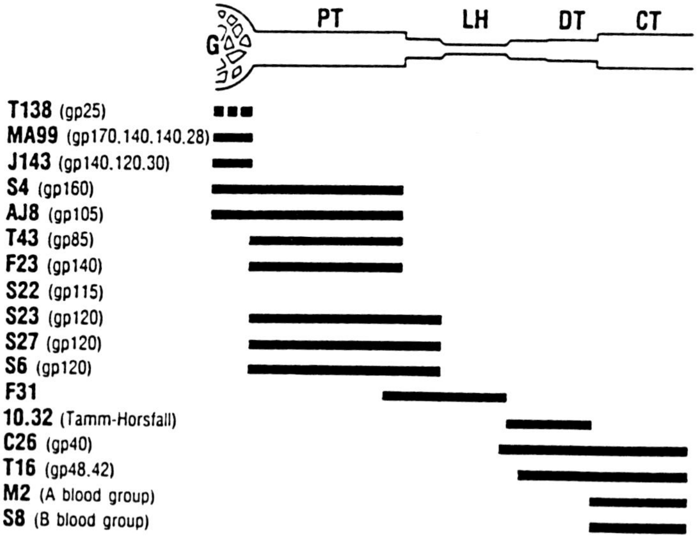

Fig. 4. Antigenic map of human nephron. Bar indicates site of binding of each monoclonal antibody as determined by immunohistochemistry on frozen kidney sections. Immunochemical characterization of each defined antigen is indicated, for example gp25 is glycoprotein with molecular weight of 25,000. S22, for which no bar is shown, does not bind to normal kidney sections but it does bind to some renal cancers. PT = proximal tubule; LH = loop of Henle; DT = distal tubule; CT = collecting tubule; G = glomerulus [from 39, with permission].

Acknowledgements

The author wishes to express his gratitude to Landis Griffeth, MD, PhD and Michael Welch, PhD for providing information concerning PET imaging. In addition, John G. McAfee, MD provided considerable information concerning ongoing investigations with monoclonal antibodies and the kidney.

References

1 Winter CC: Discussion. J Urol 1963;90:656.

2 Taplin GV, Meredith OM, Kade H, et al: The radioisotope renogram. J Lab Clin Med 1956;48:886.

3 Winter CC, Nordyke RA, Tubis M: Clinical experience with a new test agent for the radioisotope renogram: Sodium ortho-iodohippurate-^{131}I (hippuran-^{131}I). J Urol 1961;85:92.

4 Haynie TP, Nofal MM, Carr EA Jr, et al: Scintillation scanning of the kidney and radioiodinated contrast media. Clin Res 1960;8:288.

5 Schlegel JU, O'Dell RM, Izenstouk JL: Importance of stop flow to kidney scans. J Nucl Med 1963;4:320.

6 Wenzl JE, Tauxe WN, Hunt JC: A single injection technique for renal photoscanning with ortho-iodohippurate. A preliminary report. Mayo Clin Proc 1963;38:313.

7 Rosenthall L: Ortho-iodohippurate-^{131}I kidney scanning in renal failure. Radiology 1966;87;298.

8 Freeman LM, Goldman SM, Shaw R, et al: Kidney visualization with ^{131}I-orthoiodohippurate in patients with renal insufficiency. J Nucl Med 1969;10:545.

9 Borghgraef RRM, Pitts RF: Distribution of chlormerodrin (neohydrin) in the tissues of rat and dog. J Clin Invest 1956;35:31.

10 Blau M, Bender MA: A radiomercury (^{203}Hg)-labeled neohydrin. A new agent for brain tumor localization (abstract). J Nucl Med (special convention issue), June 1959, p 35.

11 McAfee JG, Wagner HN Jr: Visualization of renal parenchyma. Scintiscanning with ^{203}Hg neohydrin. Radiology 1960;75:820.

12 Sodee DB: A new scanning isotope. Mercury-197: A preliminary report. J Nucl Med 1963;4:335.

13 Rosenthall L: Applications of the gamma ray scintillation camera to dynamic studies in man. Radiology 1966;86:634.

14 Powell MR, Anger HO: Blood flow visualization with the scintillation camera. J Nucl Med 1966;7:729.

15 Raynaud C, Degrez A, Kellershohn C: Measurement of renal mercury uptake by external counting: separate function testing of each kidney. J Urol 1968;99:248.

16 Arnold RW, Subramanian G, McAfee JG, et al: Comparison of ^{99m}Tc complexes for renal imaging. J Nucl Med 1975;16:357.

17 Davison J, Jones A, Orvig C, et al: A new class of oxotechnetium (+5) chelate complexes containing a Tc ON252 core. Inorgan Chem 1981;20:1629.

18 Fritzberg AR, Kasina S, Eshima D, et al: Synthesis and biologic evaluation of Tc-99m-MAG$_3$ as a hippuran replacement. J Nucl Med 1986;27:111.

19 Williams ED, Parker C, Rankin D, et al: Multiple-section tomography of the kidney: a clinical evaluation. Br J Radiol 1986;59:975.

20 Rado JP, Bamos C, Tako J, et al: Radioisotope renography during finosemide (lasix) diuresis. Nuklearmedizin 1968;7:212.

21 O'Reilly PH: Current status of diuretic renography. Nucl Med Annu 1987;8:173.

22 Oei HY, Gekyskes GG, Dorhourt Mees EJ, et al: Captopril induced renographic alteration in renal artery stenosis. J Nucl Med 1984;25:36.

23 Sfakianakis GN, Sfakianakis E, Bourgoignie J: Renal scintigraphy following angioinsin-converting enzyme inhibition in the diagnosis of renovascular hypertension (captopril scintigraphy). Nucl Med Annu 1988;9:125.

24 Clorius JH, Dreikorn K, Zelt J, et al: Posture-induced disturbance of pertechnetate flow and ^{123}I-iodohippurate transport in some renal graft recipients with hypertension. J Nucl Med 1980;21:829.

25 Clorius J, Schmidlin P: The exercise renogram. A new approach documents renal involvement in systemic hypertension. J Nucl Med 1983;24:104.

26 Kawamura J, Itoh H, Yoshida O, et al: In vivo estimation of renal volume using a rotating gamma camera for ^{99m}Tc-dimercaptosuccinic acid renal imaging. Eur J Nucl Med 1984;9:168.

27 Yano Y, Anger HO: Visualization of heart and kidneys in animals with short-lived ^{82}Rb and the positron scintillation camera. J Nucl Med 1968;9:413.

28 Tamaki N, Rabito CA, Alpert NM: Serial analysis of renal blood flow by positron tomography with rubidium-82. Am J Physiol 1986;251:H1024.

29 Tamaki N, Alpert NM, Rabito CA, et al: The effect of captopril on renal blood flow in renal artery stenosis assessed by positron tomography with rubidium-82. Hypertension 1988;11:217.

30 Selwyn AP, Shea MJ, Foale R, et al: Regional myocardial and organ blood flow after myocardial infarction: Application of the microsphere principle in man. Circulation 1986;73:433.

31 Peters PE, Ter-Pogossian MM, Rockoff ML, et al: Measurement of renal blood flow by means of radioactive water labeled with oxygen-15; in Radionuclides in Nephrology. Blanfox MD, Funck-Brentano JL (eds): New York, Grune & Stratton, 1972.

32 Shelton ME, Green MA, Mathias CJ, et al: Measurement of regional blood flow using copper-PTSM and positron emission tomography. J Nucl Med 1989;30:807.

33 Paul R, Johansson R, Kellokumpo-Lehtinen PL, et al: Tumor localization with ^{18}F-2-fluoro-2-deoxy-*D*-glucose: comparative autoradiography, glucose-6-phosphatase histochemistry, and histology of renal implanted sarcoma of the rat. Res Exp Med 1985;185:87.

34 Schuhmacher J, Maier-Borst W, Wellman HN: Liver and Kidney imaging with ^{68}Ga-labeled dihydroxyanthranquinones. J Nucl Med 1980;21:983.

35 Hunt FC: Phenolic aminocarboxylic acids as gallium-binding radiopharmaceuticals. Nuklearmedizin 1984;23:123.

36 Clelland CC, Giles KD, Farley TD, et al: The intravenous distribution of a radiolabeled, potentially useful cluster ion of copper and penicillamine. Physiol Chem Phys Med NMR 1986;18:37.

37 Yamashita M, Inaba T, Kawase Y, et al: Quantitative measurement of renal function using Ga-68-EDTA. Tohuku J Exp Med 1988;155:207.

38 Schelstraete K, Deman J, Vermeulen FL, et al: Kinetics of ^{13}N-ammonia incorporation in human tumors. Nucl Med Commun 1985;6:461.

39 Bander N: Monoclonal antibodies: State of the art. J Urol 1987;137:603.

40 Klotz LH, Bander NH, Thompson R, et al: Staging and monitoring of renal cell carcinoma by serum assay for proximal tubular antigen (abstract). J Urol 1985;133:155.

Leonard M. Freeman, MD, Henry and Lucy Moses Hospital Division,
111 East 210th Street, Bronx, NY 10461-2490 (USA)

Blaufox MD, Hollenberg NK, Raynaud C (eds): Radionuclides in Nephro-Urology.
Contrib Nephrol. Basel, Karger, 1990, vol 79, pp 99–102

Abnormal Renal Mobility: Radionuclide Features and Clinical Relevance

P.H. O'Reilly, A.J. Pollard[1]

Departments of Urology and Nuclear Medicine, Stepping Hill Hospital, Stockport, Cheshire, UK

Abnormal renal mobility (nephroptosis) has long been a debatable entity in clinical urological practice. Indeed, its correction by nephropexy has been described as an 'ineffective operation for an imaginary disease' [1]. Such conclusions have, however, usually been based on inexact data from inaccurate methods of assessment. Since the advent of radionuclide renal scanning, the syndrome and significance of abnormal renal mobility have become clearer. Our experience with this problem is described here.

Patients and Methods

During a 24-month period, 11 patients (10 females, aged 25–59, mean 39; 1 male aged 32) undergoing urological evaluation were found to have significant degrees of abnormal renal mobility. The right kidney was affected in all cases. Abnormal renal mobility was only diagnosed on strict criteria (see below) and minor degrees of vertical movement were not considered abnormal. The female patients presented with right loin or right upper quadrant abdominal pain; all had normal intravenous urograms except one, who had dilatation of the right renal pelvis suggestive of idiopathic hydronephrosis. The male patient had bilateral idiopathic hydronephrosis, discovered during evaluation of a urinary tract infection.

Erect ^{123}I–hippuran renography was performed by standard technique using 17.5 MBq of the radiopharmaceutical and a Scintronix gamma camera with dedicated computer system [2]. ^{99m}Tc-dimercaptosuccinic acid (DMSA) scanning was performed using 70 MBq of the radiopharmaceutical and scanning in the erect and supine positions as necessary at 3 h. Split renal function from the hippuran study was calculated in the usual way [2]. Split function from the DMSA study was calculated in the erect position by taking the geometric mean of anterior and posterior images, and in the supine position by using posterior images only. Where obstruction was suspected, erect and supine diuresis renograms were performed giving the diuretic at 20 min into the test.

[1] Thanks are due to all the staff of the Nuclear Medicine Department at Stepping Hill Hospital.

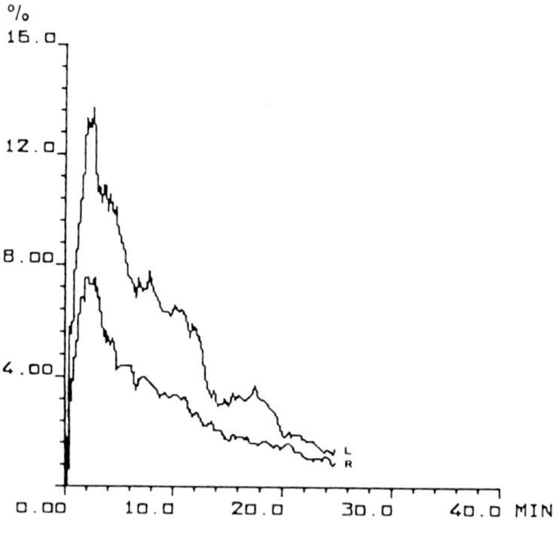

Fig. 1. Composite of ^{123}I-hippuran renogram curve (left) and DMSA renal images (right). The renogram curve shows a normal left curve, and a 'miniaturised' right curve but with normal time to peak and elimination phase. The DMSA scans show apparent small right kidney on erect image (top), normal right kidney on supine image (middle), and rotational prolapse downwards and forwards on oblique image (bottom). The 'miniaturised' renogram curve is the result of erect imaging of a functionally normal nephroptotic kidney viewed end-on by the camera.

Results

Radionuclide Studies

On initial erect ^{123}I-hippuran renography, all cases showed an apparently small right kidney with reduced renal function (range 27–41%, mean 33%). In 9 cases, the curve shapes were normal and nonobstructed, but were reduced in size or *miniaturised.* Similar small right renal images were seen on erect ^{99m}Tc-DMSA scans. However, if split renal function was derived by taking the geometric mean of anterior and posterior images in the erect position, it was normal (range 46–53%, mean 48%). Oblique erect imaging demonstrated the right kidney to be prolapsing both downwards and forwards, rotating through an AP axis with the lower pole projecting anteriorly, thus accounting for the *apparently* small right renal image, artefactually low function and miniaturised renogram curve. In contrast, supine DMSA images showed equal and normal appearances on left and right (fig. 1). In the female patient with urographic renal pelvic dilatation, and in the male patient, standard ^{123}I-hippuran renogram curves were obstructed.

Clinical Results

Of the 9 nonobstructed patients, 4 had mild pain only and no further action was required. Five patients had right nephropexy to fix the kidney in its normal position. All had normal post-operative DMSA studies. In 3 cases, lasting relief of symptoms was achieved (follow-up $>$ 2 years). In 2 cases, sibling girls, right loin pain returned 9 months after surgery, in spite of normal position, function and drainage in the right kidney.

The female patient with renal pelvic dilatation had an obstructed erect diuresis renogram. When repeated supine, there was no obstruction. An assumption was made that the obstruction was posturally associated with the renal mobility. At operation there was no evidence of intrinsic uretero-pelvic junction obstruction and simple renal fixation alone was performed. DMSA scanning on the 5th post-operative day was normal. However, ^{123}I-hippuran renography 5 days after this showed obstruction and reduced split renal function. Excretion urography suggested gross ureteropelvic junction obstruction. A double-J indwelling ureteric split was introduced cystoscopically, and later a dismembered pyeloplasty performed. Post-operative diuresis renography was unobstructed with restored normal split function.

The male patient with bilateral hydronephrosis on urography had nonobstructive ^{99m}Tc-DTPA supine renograms elsewhere. Erect ^{123}I-hippuran renograms showed right nephroptosis and an obstructive curve. It was judged that the abnormal renal mobility was converting nonobstructed hydronephrosis to obstructed hydronephrosis. Nephropexy with dismembered pyeloplasty were performed. Post-operative DMSA scan and diuresis renography were normal.

Discussion

Doubts about the significance of abnormal renal mobility and the indications for surgical correction have been fuelled by inaccurate diagnosis, poor surgical results and the absence of reliable objective tests for pre-and post-operative assessment. The increasing sophistication of renal imaging modalities, especially radionuclide scintigraphy, have increased our knowledge of renal structure and function. The cases described here first came to light because we perform hippuran renography in the erect position to include the normal hydrostatic component of urine transport during evaluation of upper tract urodynamics. Thus the syndrome of artefactually small right renal images apparently reduced renal function and miniaturised renogram curves in patients with right loin or upper right abdominal pain evolved. Supine studies miss such renal mobility. The phenomenon is not very common, only 11 cases being found in the past 2 years; minor irrelevant degrees of vertical movement are much more frequent. However, even these few cases allow several conclusions to be drawn.

First, when a significant degree of vertical renal movement is accompanied by rotational movement in an AP axis, renal pain may be produced. The exact mechanism is unknown, but tension on the renal pedicle or renal vein torsion have been suggested [L. Glickman, unpubl. data].

Secondly, abnormal renal mobility may produce erroneous split renal function results during erect renography. Investigators should be aware of this possibility, especially where functional estimate and scintigram appearances seem to contradict other data such as urography, and where surgical decision-making depends on the results of renal function data.

Third, the role of surgery must be examined critically. In many cases, the degree of discomfort will not justify surgery. If renal fixation is considered necessary, it will cure some patients, but the mechanism of pain production and its relief are unknown, and the possibility of recurrence of symptoms at a later date must be borne in mind to avoid overoptimistic expectations in both surgeon and patient.

Fourth, where obstruction coexists with abnormal mobility, a causal relationship should not be assumed. One of our cases had intermittent hydronephrosis as well as nephroptosis. Correction of the latter did nothing to eradicate the former, and secondary surgery was required. Another case had gross nonobstructive dilatation, converted to obstructive hydronephrosis by the renal movement. Obstructive conditions occurring in association with nephroptosis should be evaluated as independent entities, and may require synchronous treatment.

References

1 McWhinnie DL, Hamilton DNH: The rise and fall of surgery for the floating kidney. Br Med J 1984;288:845–847.

2 Hastings DL, Prescott MC: Protocols of procedures; in O'Reilly PH, Shields RA, Testa HJ (eds): Nuclear Medicine in Urology and Nephrology, ed 2. London, Butterworth, 1986, pp. 77–88.

P.H. O'Reilly, MD, Departments of Urology and Nuclear Medicine,
Stepping Hill Hospital, Stockport SK2 7JE, Cheshire (UK)

Blaufox MD, Hollenberg NK, Raynaud C (eds): Radionuclides in Nephro-Urology.
Contrib Nephrol. Basel, Karger, 1990, vol 79, pp 103–107

The Uses and Interpretation of Modified Diuresis Renography[1]

S.M. Upsdell, H.J. Testa, R.S. Lawson, R.N.P. Carroll, E.C. Edwards

Departments of Nuclear Medicine and Urology, Manchester Royal Infirmary, Manchester, UK

Diuresis renography is widely accepted in clinical practice for the investigation of dilatation of the upper urinary tracts. However, despite over 10 years' experience with this technique, equivocal results are still obtained in up to 15% of cases [1]. For several years we have employed a modified method of diuresis renography in which the diuretic is given 15 min *before* the radiopharmaceutical, which we refer to as 'F minus 15' (F – 15) renography [2]. The rationale behind this method was that the maximum urinary flow rates occurring 15 min after the administration of frusemide [3] would be more likely to produce washout in grossly dilated systems, or to reveal obstruction in systems that only obstruct at high urine flow rates, than standard diuresis renography.

The purpose of this study was to investigate the effect of early administration of frusemide on the renogram curve and to establish the indications for its use. In addition to its diuretic action, frusemide produces changes in renal haemodynamics [4, 5]. This study also investigated changes in renal plasma flow during the first 2 min of the renogram and their effect on relative function estimates.

Materials and Methods

We studied 112 adult patients aged between 16 and 54 years (mean 39). All patients underwent both standard diuresis renography and F – 15 renography on the same day. All renograms were performed in the sitting position with the gamma camera placed posteriorly. Renography was performed using 0.2 MBq/kg of ^{123}I-hippuran. Frusemide was given intravenously in a dose of 0.5 mg/kg at approximately 20 min into the renogram in standard renography and 15 min *before* the test in F – 15 renography. The F – 15 renogram usually followed immediately after the standard renogram so that the same dose of frusemide was

[1] Supported by the North West of England Kidney Research Association.

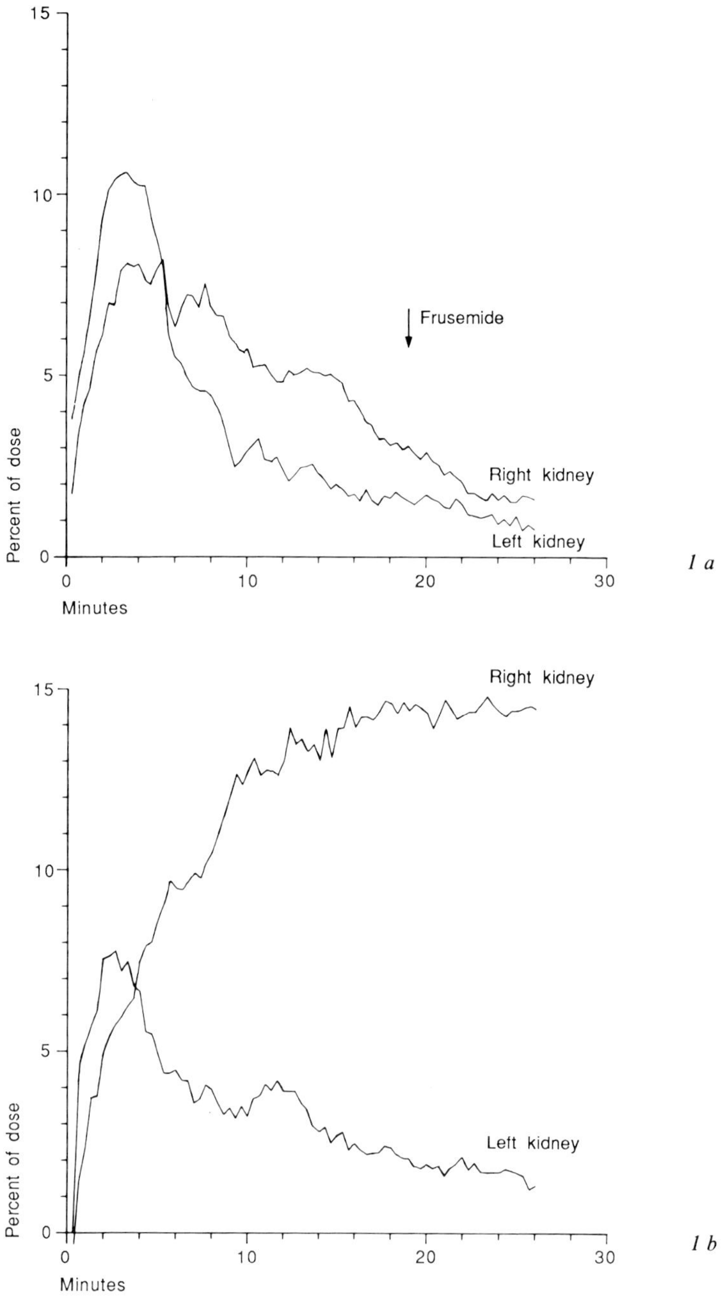

Fig. 1. a A standard diuresis renogram in patient with right-sided loin pain and radiographic dilatation showing equivocal washout on right side. *b* F – 15 renogram on the same day showing obstructed pattern on the right side.

used for both tests. Where necessary, the F – 15 renogram was corrected for any background activity remaining from the first test.

The renograms were assessed for 2 min uptake, time to peak, relative function and pattern of elimination. Two minute uptake was defined as the percentage of the injected dose in the kidney at 2 min after injection. This was calculated from the background subtracted counts in the kidney region of interest during the 20-second frame with its end point at 2 min. The 2 min uptake of hippuran has been shown by several authors to correlate well with renal plasma flow [6–8] and this relationship has been confirmed by previous studies in our department. Time to peak was defined as the time from injection until the peak of the renogram curve and was only calculated in those kidneys with an easily definable peak. Relative function of the kidneys was calculated from the integral of the renogram curve from 1 min after injection until the peak (or 5 min, whichever was the earlier) expressed as a percentage of the total area under both curves. The incidence of equivocal patterns of elimination was established for both methods of diuresis renography. The Student's t test for paired data was used for statistical analysis.

Results

A significant increase in 2 min uptake was demonstrated in the F – 15 renograms ($p < 0.001$). 116 kidneys were suitable for time to peak calculations and there was a highly significant decrease in the time to peak in the F – 15 renogram ($p < 0.001$). The relative function of the left kidney was compared in 112 patients and there was no significant difference in this estimate with the two methods of diuresis renography. Equivocal washout was seen in 19 cases using standard diuresis renography. F – 15 renography clarified 16 of these cases with 10 cases showing an obstructed pattern (fig. 1) and 6 cases a nonobstructed pattern. This left only 3 equivocal cases.

Discussion

Frusemide is known to increase renal blood flow in both animals and humans [4, 5] and this has also been shown in this study by the increase in 2 min uptake seen in the F – 15 renograms. The increase in urinary flow rates achieved by giving frusemide 15 min before the test results in a reduced time to peak in the F – 15 renogram and a rapid washout pattern so that washout from the kidney is usually complete by 20 min. Despite alterations in renal plasma flow and a reduction in the amount of data available before the peak of the renogram, relative function estimates are not significantly changed in F – 15 renography. Comparison of relative function estimates by standard diuresis renography and F – 15 renography is therefore valid and these two methods can be used to evaluate relative function on sequential renograms.

A normal F – 15 renogram should have rapid uptake of the tracer, an early peak and rapid washout (fig. 2). If there is any departure from this

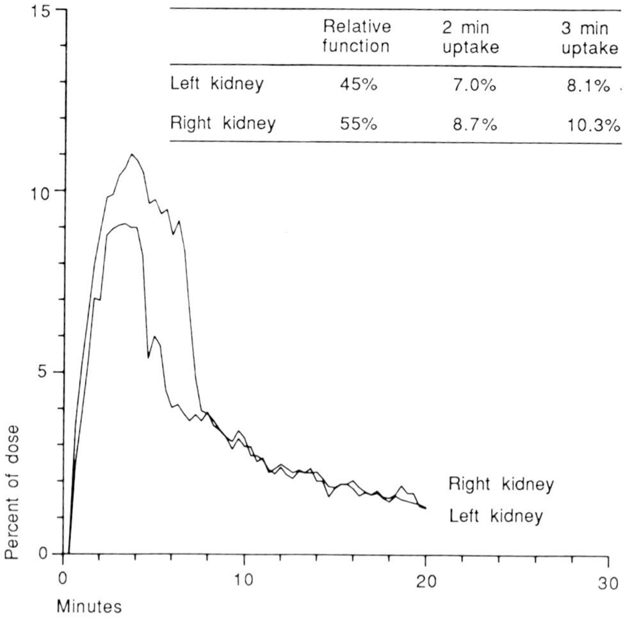

	Relative function	2 min uptake	3 min uptake
Left kidney	45%	7.0%	8.1%
Right kidney	55%	8.7%	10.3%

2 *a*

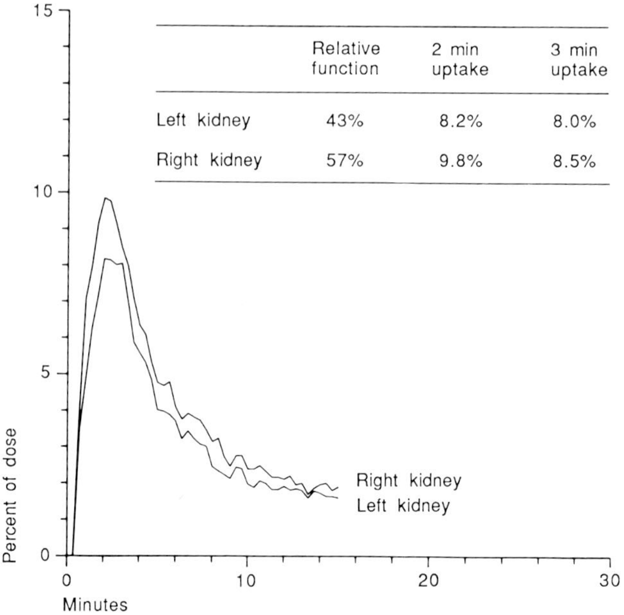

	Relative function	2 min uptake	3 min uptake
Left kidney	43%	8.2%	8.0%
Right kidney	57%	9.8%	8.5%

2 *b*

Fig. 2. a Standard renogram. Time to peak 3.4 min left, 3.6 min right. *b* F – 15 renogram on the same day showing a decrease in the time to peak (2.0 min left, 2.0 min right), rapid washout and increased 2 min uptake.

normal curve, further tests such as perfusion pressure flow studies or repeat renography are indicated.

The rate of equivocal results from standard diuresis renography was 17% in this series. The F−15 renogram reduced this rate to 3%. In a recently completed study into the long-term follow-up of patients investigated by F−15 renography [unpubl. data], we have shown that the results of this test are reliable in the evaluation of the upper urinary tract, and that clinical management decisions based on these results have been correct. It is now our policy to perform F−15 renography in all renographically or clinically equivocal cases.

References

1 O'Reilly PH, Testa HJ, Lawson RS, et al: Diuresis renography in equivocal urinary tract obstruction. Br J Urol 1984;56:84.

2 English PJ, Testa HJ, Lawson RS, et al: Modified method of diuresis renography for the assessment of equivocal pelviureteric obstruction. Br J Urol 1987;59:10–14.

3 Upsdell SM, Leeson SM, Brooman PJC, et al: Diuretic induced urinary flow rates at varying clearances and their relevance to the performance and interpretation of diuresis renography. Br J Urol 1988;61:14–18.

4 Brater DC: Pharmacodynamic considerations in the use of diuretics. Annu Rev Pharmacol Toxicol 1983;23:45–62.

5 Weiner IM, Mudge GH: Diuretics and other agents employed in the mobilisation of oedema fluid; in Gilman AF, Goodman LS (eds): The Pharmacological Basis of Therapeutics, ed 7. London, Saunders, 1985, pp. 896–897.

6 Schlegel JU, Hamway SA: Individual renal plasma flow determination in 2 minutes. J Urol 1976;116:282–285.

7 Shames DM, Korobkin M: A simple technique for measuring relative renal blood flow. J Nucl Med 1976;17:876–879.

8 Fine EJ, Axelrod M, Gorkin J, et al: Measurement of effective renal plasma flow: A comparison of methods. J Nucl Med 1987;23:1393–1400.

S.M. Upsdell, FRCS, Department of Nuclear Medicine, Manchester Royal Infirmary, Oxford Road, Manchester M13 9WL (UK)

Blaufox MD, Hollenberg NK, Raynaud C (eds): Radionuclides in Nephro-Urology.
Contrib Nephrol. Basel, Karger, 1990, vol 79, pp 108–112

Prospective Evaluation of Radionuclide Monitoring in Renal Transplantation

Henrik S. Thomsen, Peter Bartram, Keld Hvid-Jacobsen, Steen Levin Nielsen[1]

Departments of Nuclear Medicine and Nephrology, Herlev Hospital, University of Copenhagen, Herlev, Denmark

Radionuclide monitoring of renal grafts has been performed routinely following all transplantations (approx. 600 cases) for more than 13 years. From the start of the program, radionuclide monitoring included ^{99m}Tc-pertechnetate angiography of the graft and ^{131}I-hippuran renography on gamma camera. The first examination is done within 36 h after operation and afterwards routinely 3 times a week, and if indicated at other times. Since 1985, renography has been performed until discharge (or graft removal), whereas dynamic radionuclide angiography has been done only until the clinical situation has stabilized and thereafter in case of clinical or renographic suspicion of graft dysfunction [1]. For description we use a simple qualitative grading. By visual inspection of the normalized first passage curve of the intravenous bolus it is determined whether the graft has a well-defined flow peak (=normal perfusion), poorly defined flow peak (=reduced perfusion) or no flow peak (=severely reduced perfusion) (fig. 1). The renal function as judged from the renograms is described by a grading system [2], where grade 0 depicts the normal renogram and grade 5 the flat curve (fig. 2). The qualitative estimations may seem rough but for clinical purposes they have turned out to be sufficient [1]. For example, it has enabled us to demonstrate objectively that immunosuppression with 'high dose' ciclosporin A in ischemic grafts correlates with high frequency of nephrotoxicity [1, 3, 4]. After a 3-year period where the present monitoring and description system was interpreted in close cooperation with the nephrologists in the daily routine, we found it valuable to study its effect on the clinical decisions.

[1] Other members of the study group included senior residents and consultants at the two departments.

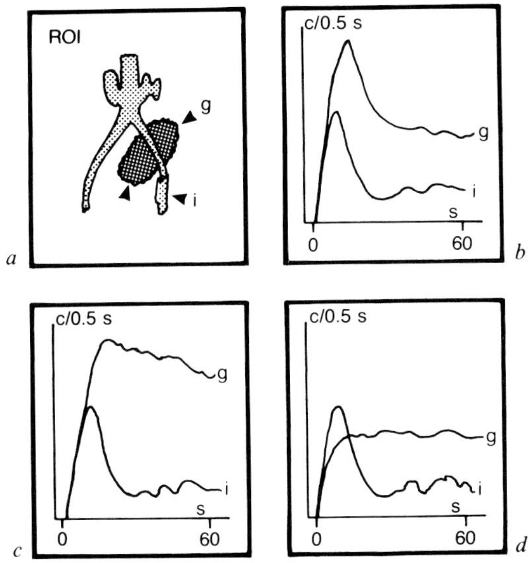

Fig. 1. Drawing *(a)* with regions of interest *(*arrowheads*)* over graft (g) without the underlying iliac artery and over the iliac artery (i). Histogram *(b)* showing a well-defined flow peak on both the graft and the iliac artery. Histograms from the graft region of interest with a poorly defined flow peak *(c)* and without a flow peak *(d)* despite well-defined flow peaks on the iliac histograms.

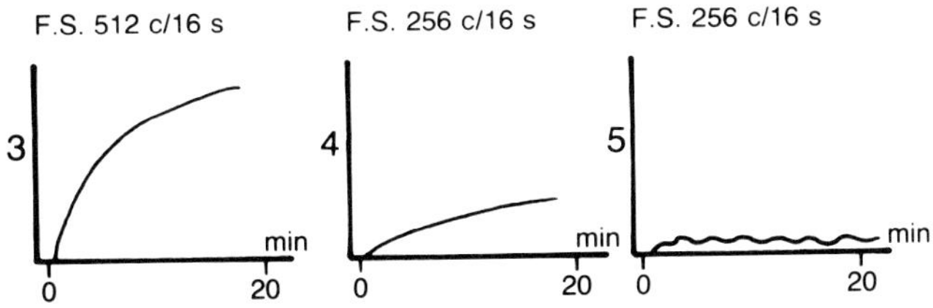

Fig. 2. ^{131}I-hippuran renograms from renal allograft graded according to the function of the graft: Grade 0 is from a graft with normal glomerular filtration rate. Grades 1 through 4 show the pattern of renograms when function decreases. The flat renogram, grade 5, indicates nearly abolished function.

Methods

During a 13-month period a total of 34 kidneys have been transplanted. Following each radionuclide examination during the first 5 postoperative weeks the nephrologist on duty prospectively answers a questionnaire concerning clinical suspicion before and what consequence was taken of the result of the examination. It should be noted whether nothing (unchanged circumstances or confirmation of progress) was done, another diagnostic procedure (e.g. ultrasonography, percutaneous graft biopsy, i.v. urography, pyelography, arteriography) was requested, or a medical (e.g. increased steroid treatment, change of dose of ciclosporin A) or a surgical intervention was performed, and whether biochemical data and/or clinical symptoms/signs also pointed towards a complication. At the following radionuclide examination it was checked whether the questionnaire had been filled out after the previous examination. After the patient's discharge the record was reviewed; it was noted whether the supplementary diagnostic procedure or the intervention had been done and the result/consequence of the procedure/intervention was registered.

Renography was performed after intravenous injection of 10–12 MBq ^{131}I-hippuran using a Siemens ZLC scintillation camera coupled to a Siemens scintiview computer. Eighty-four frames were taken with 16 s intervals. Background subtraction used a symmetrical region of interest placed in the contralateral site of pelvis. Graft perfusion was studied prior to renography by a bolus injection of 370 MBq ^{99m}Tc-pertechnetate into a cubital vein. The equipment was the same as for renography, 127 frames of 0.5 s were obtained. Two regions of interest were chosen, the one being the graft without underlying major vessels and the other the iliac artery. The iliac histograms were used to ascertain a proper bolus injection, shown by a well-defined peak on the iliac artery histogram and a $T_{1/2}$ of the down slope of less than 10 s. In that case, the graft curve was graded. After the patient's discharge both the renograms and the first passage curves were re-evaluated. A complication was suspected if the flow peak disappeared and/or the function as judged from the renograms fell significantly (e.g. from grade 2 to a intermediate position between grade 2 and grade 3 or more).

Results

A total of 300 radionuclide studies (median 10, range 1–16) were performed in the 34 consecutive patients. At the review of the records no unregistered consequence was found. The review of radionuclide curves was in agreement with the result of the daily routine. In 7 patients the postoperative course was uneventful: they had a total of 60 radionuclide examinations. In the remaining 27 patients, 32 complications were suspected by the radionuclide examination (table 1); in only 4 instances was it based on one examination, whereas in the other 28 cases it was the change in grading. At or following all 21 interventions, occurrence of a complication was verified. No registered complication remained undetected by the radionuclide studies. The effect of rejection treatment could be confirmed at the subsequent examination in 8 of the 11 episodes. In 29 instances the radionuclide examinations showed major progress, for example the function as judged from the renograms improved a degree or more or the flow peak recurred.

Table 1. Routine radionuclide examination(s) indicating a complication and consequence

Radionuclide examination(s) indicate(s) a complication	Biochemical and/or clinical signs/symptoms of a complication	Consequence		Instances
		another diagnostic procedure performed	medical and/or surgical intervention	
Yes	no	yes	yes	3
		yes	no	7
		no	yes	5
Yes	yes	yes	yes	8
		yes	no	4
		no	yes	5
No	yes	yes	yes	0
		yes	no	6
		no	yes	0

Discussion

The present study shows that in a small transplantation center, radionuclide monitoring of renal grafts is of great importance. When the examination is incorporated in the routine evaluation at least 3 times a week and the result of the examination is presented in a simple way, a strong confidence is obtained, and the impact on the nephrologist's clinical decision is high. As regards complications, a sensitivity of 100% and a specificity of 66% were reached. A better specificity might have been obtained if we had refined our simple evaluation of the curves with quantitation of perfusion indices or transit times. Among the 300 studies, 13% were correct-positive and 7% were false-positive. At first glance this seem a low cost/benefit ratio, but one may not underestimate the value of the 80% correct-negative studies confirming progress or unchanged circumstances in a group of patients who are at risk of too many serious complications in the early postoperative course. Furthermore, the change in each patient is most frequently of importance, increasing the value of the repeated investigations. As a matter of fact, in 28 instances it was the change that indicated a complication and in 29 instances the change indicated significant improvement bringing the number of diagnostic examinations up to 118 (39%). In nonfunctioning grafts radionuclide examination is often the only available functional parameter for graft perfusion and tubular uptake. It is concluded that radionuclide monitoring is very valuable in the early stages of renal transplantation.

References

1 Thomsen HS, Løkkegaard H, Nielsen SL, et al: Postoperative radionuclide monitoring of renal allografts on triple therapy. Dan Med Bull 1988;35:395–397.

2 Thomsen HS, Dorph S, Mygind T, et al: The transplanted kidney. Diagnostic and interventional radiology. Acta Radiol Diagn 1985;26:353–367.

3 Thomsen HS, Munck O: Nephrotoxicity of ciclosporin in transplanted kidneys demonstrated with the ^{99m}Tc perfusion studies. Contr Nephrol. Basel, Karger, 1987. Vol 56, pp 159–162.

4 Thomsen HS, Nielsen SL: Triple therapy and initial renal graft perfusion. Dan Med Bull 1988;35:393–395.

Henrik S, Thomsen, MD, Department of Diagnostic Radiology 54 E2,
Herlev Hospital, University of Copenhagen, Herlev Ringvej 75,
DK–2730 Herlev (Denmark)

Blaufox MD, Hollenberg NK, Raynaud C (eds): Radionuclides in Nephro-Urology. Contrib Nephrol. Basel, Karger, 1990, vol 79, pp 113–117

Measurements of ^{99m}Tc-MAG_3 Uptake in Renal Transplant Recipients

H.Y. Oei[a], *S. Surachno*[b], *J.M. Wilmink*[b], *J.B. van der Schoot*[a]

Departments of [a]Nuclear Medicine and [b]Nephrology, Academic Medical Center, Amsterdam, The Netherlands

Mercaptoacetyltriglycine (MAG_3) is a new, technetium-labelled, mainly tubular excreted agent, which is expected to replace hippuran (OIH) in many clinical applications. Although the clearance of MAG_3 is approximately 60% of the OIH clearance, studies comparing both agents for routine examinations in patients with a variety of renal disorders showed identical results. The physiological properties of MAG_3 which are equivalent to OIH, and its availability as technetium-labelled kit preparation, make this pharmaceutical very attractive [2, 4, 7–9].

In this study we performed serial measurements of 10-min uptake during standardized renography in two groups of renal transplant patients using ^{123}I-OIH and ^{99m}Tc-MAG_3 respectively. The 10-min uptake value measured in this way depends on the renal blood flow and the capacity of the tubules to extract the compound from the blood, and therefore we use the abbreviations HUC_{10} and MUC_{10} (hippuran, MAG_3 uptake capacity). Our group as well as others have shown the value of such measurements for the monitoring during the early posttransplant period [1, 3, 5, 6]. The aim of this study was to evaluate whether MAG_3 can replace OIH for this purpose.

Patients and Methods

Data were obtained from two groups of patients (table 1): group 1 consists of 24 patients, 14 male and 10 female, aged 22–68 (44 ± 13) years, was studied with 20 MBq ^{123}I-OIH, and group 2, consisting of 33 patients, 16 male and 17 female, aged 20–68 (42 ± 14) years, was studied using 50 MBq ^{99m}Tc-MAG_3. All patients were initially treated with ciclosporin and low dosage prednisone. On the basis of the clinical course each group was divided into three subgroups: (a) uneventful course (UC); (b) ciclosporin toxicity (CT), and (c) acute rejection (AR). These diagnoses were made retrospectively based on the clinical signs and symptoms and were supported by fine needle aspiration cytology and the response to the

Table 1. Number of patients in groups and subgroups studied

Clinical course	Group 1[1]	Group 2[1]
Uneventful course	11 (2)	10 (7)
Ciclosporin toxicity	7 (2)	14 (5)
Acute rejection	6 (3)	9 (4)

[1]Number of patients with acute tubular necrosis in parentheses.

given therapy. The numbers in parentheses shown in table 1 indicate the number of patients in each subgroup having acute tubular necrosis (ATN), which is defined as a condition where the serum creatinine was not declining immediately after transplantation, without evidence of AR or CT. As shown in table 1, ATN occurs more frequently in group 2 patients. Patients suffering from other than the above complications were excluded from the study.

The measurement of 10-min uptake during standardized renography was described in detail in our previous publications [5, 6]. In the present study three modifications were introduced: (1) For the OIH study the injected dose was measured with the gamma camera as in the original methods; whereas for the MAG_3 study the injected dose was calculated by measuring the activity of a 10 MBq ^{99m}Tc standard· (2) The acquisition of the scintigraphic data during the whole examination was performed in 15 s frames. (3) The HUC_{10} and MUC_{10} are calculated as follows: the integral counts of kidney and bladder in the 1–10 min divided by the injected dose in counts/s. For the calculation the first minute was left out to exclude the influence of the first passage and the inaccuracy of the start of the integration.

The first examination was performed within the first 4 days after transplantation and renography was repeated with an interval of 2–5 days and also when suspicion of complications arose. Most patients underwent four examinations during the first 16 days after the transplantation using a gamma camera (Siemens LFOV or GF Maxi 400T) equipped with a low-energy all-purpose collimator and Gamma-11 computer system. The ^{99m}Tc-MAG_3 was prepared from a kit formulation supplied by Mallinckrodt Diagnostica. The labelling procedure was performed according to the prescription of the manufacturer. The labelled agent was used within 1 h after the procedure. ^{123}I-OIH was supplied by Cygne. Statistical significance was tested using the Wilcoxon or Mann-Whitney-Wilcoxon method.

Results and Discussion

The results are summarized in table 2. As shown in the first two columns the HUC_{10} and MUC_{10} values obtained from the first examination in patients with ATN are significantly lower than in patients with an immediate functioning graft. This is in accordance with our previous study using ^{131}I-OIH [6]. Although our patients were not studied with both agents, from these values obtained during the first measurement in both groups it can be assumed that the MUC_{10} is approximately two thirds of the corresponding HUC_{10}. Estimations of MAG_3 and OIH excretion have

Table 2. Range (mean ± SD) of HUC_{10} and MUC_{10} values

	Acute tubular necrosis[1]	Immediate functioning graft[1]	Uneventful course[2]			Ciclosporin toxicity[3]	Acute rejection[3]
	days 1–4	days 1–4	days 5–8	days 9–12	days 13–16		
HUC_{10}	5–30 (18 ± 10)	28–109 (60 ± 20)	105–169 (143 ± 22)	111–200 (148 ± 27)	109–224 (170 ± 40)	58–116 (73 ± 20)	12–73 (52 ± 20)
MUC_{10}	2–22 (10 ± 6)	14–78 (40 ± 16)	111–160 (136 ± 14)	124–250 (175 ± 45)	209–400 (319 ± 69)	55–103 (84 ± 16)	17–87 (63 ± 19)

[1]Value obtained in days 1–4 in arbitrary units.
[2]Percentage of the value obtained in days 1–4.
[3]Percentage of the value obtained in previous examination.

shown that the excreted amounts at 30 min postinjection are equal for both substances [7, 9]. Therefore it can be expected that bladder and kidney accumulation of both agents would also be equal after 30 min. The most probable cause of the MUC_{10} being significantly lower than the HUC_{10} value is the short integrating time, making these values more dependent on the renal clearance, which is for MAG_3 approximately 60% of the OIH clearance.

The next three columns of table 2 demonstrate the increase of both HUC_{10} and MUC_{10} in patients with a UC in the first 16 postoperative days, which we divided into four 4-day periods. The table shows the values in the last three successive periods as percentages of the values obtained during the first 4 postoperative days. As shown in table 2, both HUC_{10} and MUC_{10} increase maximally to two and four times the initial value respectively. The increase is more pronounced in patients with ATN than in patients with immediate functioning of the graft. Some of this last category patients did not show any further increase after day 8. The higher percentage increase in group 2 can probably be explained by the higher incidence of ATN in this group. In the 7 patients with postoperative ATN without other complications, MUC_{10} increased to values between 8 and 30 (16 ± 6.6) within 6–15 (10 ± 3.1) days before the graft resumed function.

In patients with oligoanuria the OIH study always shows an accumulation curve. Using MAG_3, however, we observed a flat curve in 3 patients (fig. 1). In 2 patients with oligoanuria the flat curve was obtained on the first posttransplant day; at the next examination performed, respectively on days 3 and 5, they showed an accumulation curve. In the other patient with oliguric ATN superimposed by CT, MUC_{10} decreased and the renogram

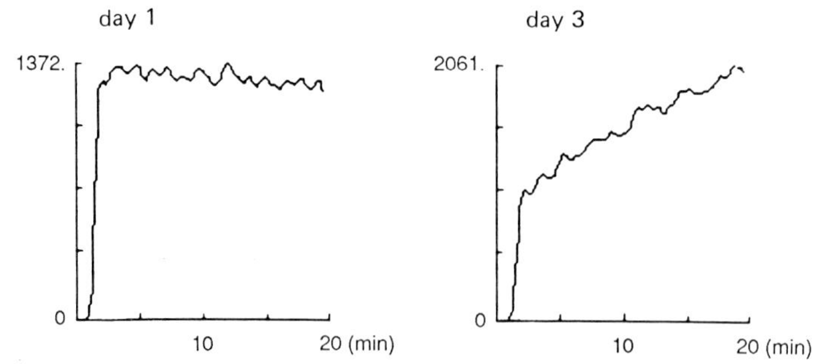

Fig. 1. MAG_3 renogram obtained from a 47-year-old cadaveric kidney recipient with oliguric ATN. He was oliguric in the first 2 weeks. The renogram obtained on the first postoperative day (left) showed a flat curve. Two days later the renogram had an accumulative type (right).

became flat on day 14. AR was excluded by biopsy and the therapy was changed into prednisone-azathioprine, after which the renogram recovered soon and the graft started functioning. A flat curve probably indicates a severe tubular injury.

Finally, the last two columns of table 2 show the uptake values during the episode of CT or AR. These values are expressed as a percentage of values obtained during the previous examination. Generally these complications were accompanied by a decrease of HUC_{10} or MUC_{10}, which was most obvious in patients with a functioning graft. Patients with ATN, whose course was disturbed by these complications, failed to show an increase of the uptake value and in this period some cases showed only a slight increase instead of the expected marked elevation. Although generally the decrease is more obvious during AR than CT, differentiating these complications on the basis of these measurements is not possible.

It can be concluded that the changes of MAG_3 uptake in renal transplant patients are equivalent to those observed in serial measurements using OIH and therefore MAG_3 can be used for the monitoring of graft function in the early posttransplant period, even in patients with oligoanuria.

References

1 Bischof-Delaloye A, Wauters JP, Delaloye B: ^{123}I-hippuran renography: accumulation and elimination indices in the long-term follow-up of renal transplants; in Joekes AM, et al (eds): Radionuclides in Nephrology. London, Academic Press, 1982, pp 284–294.

2 Bubeck B, Brandau W, Dreikorn K, et al: Clinical comparison of I-131 *o*-iodohippurate with Tc-99m CO_2-DADS-A and Tc-99m MAG_3 by simultaneous double tracer measurement. Nuc Compact 1986;17:135–138.

3 Dubovsky EV: Renal transplantation; in Tauxe WN, Dubovsky EV (eds): Nuclear Medicine in Clinical Urology and Nephrology. Norwalk, Appleton-Century-Croft, 1985, pp 233–278.

4 Jafri RA, Britton KE, Nimmon CC, et al: Technetium-99m MAG_3, a comparison with iodine-123 and iodine-131 orthoiodohippurate, in patients with renal disorders. J Nucl Med 1988;29:147–158.

5 Oei HY, Ephraim KH, Jessurun RFM: Quantitative assessment of renal transplant function on renogram performed with computer assisted gammacamera. Dial Transplant Nephrol 1975;12:441.

6 Oei HY, Jessurun RFM, Struyvenberg A: The value of renal scintigraphy for the differential diagnosis of complications after renal transplantation; in Joekes AM, et al (eds): Radionuclides in Nephrology. London, Academic Press, 1982, pp 283–288.

7 Russell CD, Thorstad B, Yester MV, et al: Comparison of technetium-99m MAG_3 with iodine-131 hippuran by a simultaneous dual channel technique. J Nucl Med 1988;29:1189–1193.

8 Schaap GH, Alferink THR, de Jong RBJ, et al: ^{99m}Tc-MAG_3: dynamic studies in patients with renal disease. Eur J Nucl Med 1988;14:28–31.

9 Taylor A Jr, Eshima D, Fritzberg AR, et al: Comparison of iodine-131 OIH and technetium-99m MAG_3 renal imaging in volunteers. J Nucl Med 1986;27:795–803.

H.Y. Oei, MD, PhD, Department of Nuclear Medicine,
University Hospital Rotterdam–Dijkzigt, Dr. Molewaterplein 40,
NL–3015 GD Rotterdam (The Netherlands)

Blaufox MD, Hollenberg NK, Raynaud C (eds): Radionuclides in Nephro-Urology.
Contrib Nephrol. Basel, Karger, 1990, vol 79, pp 118–122

Will ^{99m}Tc-MAG_3 Replace ^{131}I-OIH and ^{99m}Tc-DTPA in the Follow-Up of Renal Transplants?

E.V. Dubovsky, C.D. Russell, M.V. Yester, B.L. Thorstad, J.P. Ryan

University of Alabama in Birmingham and Birmingham Veterans Administration Medical Center, Birmingham Ala., USA

^{99m}Tc-mercaptoacetyltriglycine (MAG_3), a technetium analog of orthoidohippuran, was tested in renal graft recipients to evaluate its usefulness in the diagnosis of various complications and to compare it to the presently used radiopharmaceuticals, ^{131}I-OIH (OIH) and ^{99m}Tc-DTPA (DTPA).

Patients and Methods

Twenty-eight renal graft recipients (9 LRD, 19 cadaveric) were studied at different stages of their post-transplantation course. There were 18 males and 10 females ages 18 through 56. The diagnosis was established from the dynamic patterns of transplant complications as reported previously [1]; 13 had normally functioning grafts, 7 uncomplicated acute tubular necrosis (ATN) that resolved without therapy, 3 acute rejection (AR) and responded to OKT_3 therapy, and 1 had ciclosporin toxicity improved after dose adjustment. Of 4 patients who had a combination of problems, 2 had resolving ATN and superimposed AR confirmed by biopsy and 1 had AR with mild obstructive pattern confirmed by biopsy and ultrasound. The other patient had ATN with superimposed AR and acute and chronic inflammation of the graft and collecting system, which was diagnosed after graft nephrectomy performed 1 day later. OIH (150 μCi) and MAG_3 (5 mCi) were administered simultaneously with dual-channel acquisition and counting. Protocol consisted of: (1) sequential imaging for 27 min (120 one-second images followed by 80 twenty-second frames); (2) urine collection at 35 min with bladder imaging before and after voiding; (3) imaging of injection site to exclude infiltration; (4) urine counting, and (5) counting of a single 44-min plasma sample. From the plasma sample, effective renal plasma flow (ERPF) was calculated directly for OIH and using a proportional constant for MAG_3 [2–5]. Urine activity, corrected for residual urine volume, was divided by the activity leaving the plasma to obtain the excretory index (EI). Time-activity (T-A) curves were generated from renal regions of interest after background subtraction and time of maximum activity (peak time) was determined.

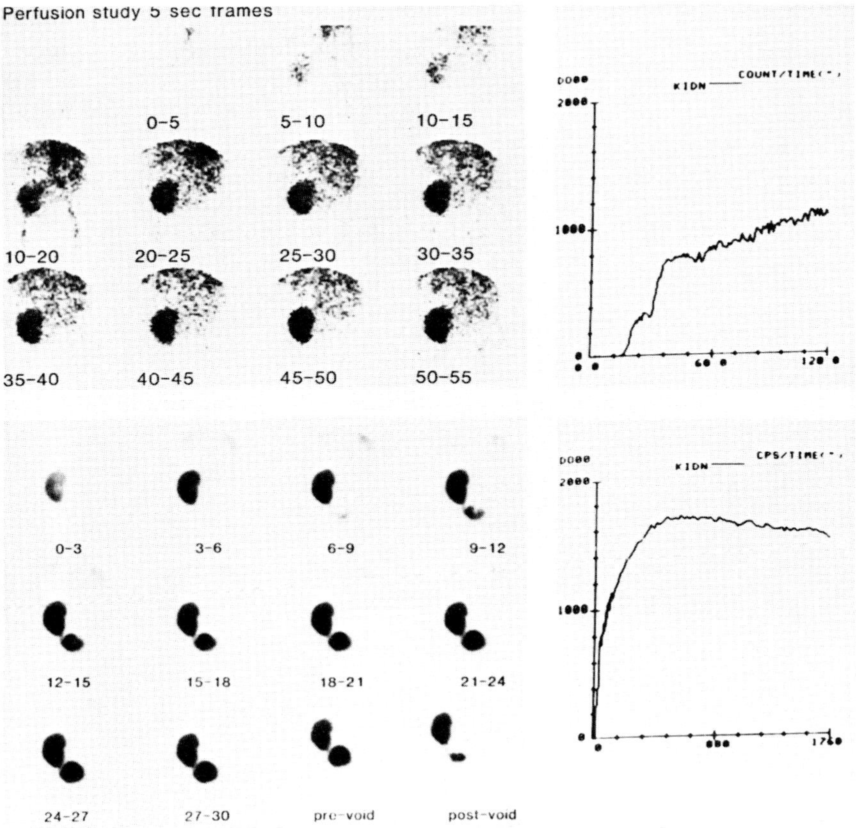

Fig. 1. Perfusion study (top) and dynamic sequence (bottom) with their respective T-A curves in a patient with resolving ATN. ERPF and EI calculated from OIH and MAG$_3$ data.

	^{131}I-OIH	^{99m}Tc-MAG$_3$
ERPF, ml/min	222	118
EI	0.44	0.48
Peak time, min	15	15

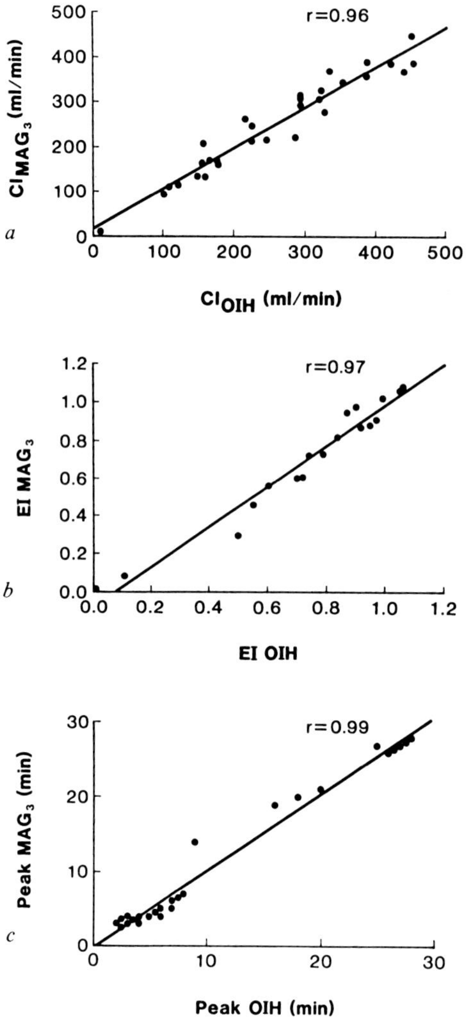

Fig. 2. Correlations of ^{99m}Tc-MAG_3 and ^{131}I-OIH quantitative data. *a* Effective renal plasma flow. *b* Excretory index. *c* Peak times.

Results

MAG_3 images were always of superior quality because of significantly higher count rate and better target-to-background ratio. Lesions, such as cortical defect, a clot in the bladder, and slight displacement of the ureter and bladder by hematoma, not seen with OIH, were visualized with MAG_3, as were the liver and native kidneys. The slightly slower washout of MAG$_3$ from the renal parenchyma led first to overestimation of cortical retention and visual underestimation of the graft function. Quantitative data (ERPF and EI) and renograms were a good guide in learning this slightly new pattern.

T-A curves (0–27 min) were similar in shape, despite the difference in slope, hence the methods based on curve analysis [6] were not affected. The perfusion curves (first 2 min), not available with OIH, were different from the ones recorded with DTPA, in which well-defined peak is usually present. MAG$_3$ perfusion curves have a steadily ascending slope caused by immediate high extraction of the agent (fig. 1), preventing the usual calculations of perfusion indices [7]. This aspect of MAG$_3$ data remains to be analyzed.

ERPF was calculated from a single 44-min blood sample [1]. Since MAG$_3$ has higher protein binding, higher plasma concentration and lower plasma clearance than OIH [3], the plasma counts of MAG$_3$ had to be multiplied by 0.563 and used instead of OIH plasma counts for ERPF calculations ($r = 0.96$) (fig. 2a) [2]. The modified ERPF and EI calculations resulted in good but not perfect correlation. An alternative approach would use the clearance of MAG$_3$ directly, which would require a change of software and reeducating the clinicians.

EI is the ratio of activity that appears in the urine to the activity leaving the blood. Low values reflect the degree of retention of activity in the collecting system (obstruction) or renal parenchyma (AR or ATN) [1]. When EI was calculated for MAG$_3$ and OIH, a linear relationship was found ($r = 0.97$) [2]. Sixteen patients were included; three had an indwelling catheter, preventing calculation of EI. Three patients with ATN, two patients with AR and two with a combination of both were anuric. In 2 patients, urine collection was incomplete (fig. 2b). Quantitative comparison of the peak time was possible in 27 patients.The correlation coefficient was 0.99 (fig. 2c). All patients were categorized correctly with the exception of a patient with a combination of ATN, AR, and infection. Use of another agent would not, however, result in a more accurate diagnosis.

Discussion

^{99m}Tc-MAG$_3$ can be substituted for OIH in the quantitative protocol of renal graft evaluation, using ERPF and EI values in a temporal manner, for differential diagnosis of various complications. MAG$_3$ images are of better quality and have more favorable dosimetry. The rapid MAG$_3$ excretion with high concentration of the agent in the parenchyma and the collecting system improves lesion detection over that of DTPA.

References

1 Dubovsky EV, Tauxe WN, Diethelm AG, et al: Dynamic patterns of kidney transplant complications using quantitative functional evolution; in Joekes AM, Constable AR, Brown NJG, et al (eds): Radionuclides in Nephrology. London, Academic Press, 1982, pp 257–262.

2 Russell CD, Thorstad B, Yester MV, et al: Quantitation of renal function with $^{99m}Tc-MAG_3$. J Nucl Med 1988;29:1931–1933.

3 Bubeck B, Brandau W, Steinbaecher M, et al: Technetium-99m-labeled renal functioning and imaging agents. II. Clinical evaluation of $^{99m}Tc-MAG_3$ (^{99m}Tc-mercaptoacetylglycylglycylglycine). Nucl Med Biol 1988;15:109–118.

4 Taylor A, Eshima D, Fritzberg AR, et al: Comparison of I-131-OIH and technetium-99m-MAG_3 renal imaging in volunteers. J Nucl Med 1986;27:795–803.

5 Jafri AR, Britton KE, Nimmon CE, et al: Technetium-99m-MAG_3, a comparison with iodine-123 and iodine-131 orthoiodohippurate in patients with renal disorders. J Nucl Med 1988;29:147–158.

6 Oei HY, Surachno S, Wilmink JM, et al: Measurements of Tc-99m-MAG_3 uptake in renal transplant. J Nucl Med 1989;30(10):3Ab–4Ab.

7 Hilson AJ, Maisey MN, Brown CB, et al: Dynamic renal transplant imaging with Tc-99m-DTPA (Sn) supplemented by a transplant perfusion index in the management of renal transplants. J Nucl Med 1978;19:994–1000.

E.V. Dubovsky, MD, Division of Nuclear Medicine, University of Alabama Hospital, 619 Nineteenth Street South, Birmingham, AL 35233 (USA)

Blaufox MD, Hollenberg NK, Raynaud C (eds): Radionuclides in Nephro-Urology.
Contrib Nephrol. Basel, Karger, 1990, vol 79, pp 123–126

The Intrarenal Kinetics of Hippuran in Acute Rejection of Renal Allograft

G. Magnusson, R. Lewander, G. Lundgren, B. Sarby, L. Svensson, S. Thornström

Department of Renal Medicine, Huddinge University Hospital, Stockholm, Sweden

Earlier experimental and clinical studies have indicated a cortical retention of hippuran of varying degree in acute rejection of renal allograft according to autoradiography [1] and scintirenography [2]. Since a similar intrarenal distribution of hippuran is also observed in ischemic injury of renal graft [3], it may be suspected that ischemia may cause the altered intrarenal kinetics of hippuran in acute rejection. The aim of this study is to answer the following two questions by means of computerized scintirenography: (a) Is there any correlation between the degree of the disturbed intrarenal kinetics of hippuran and the severity of the acute rejection? (b) To which extent do the observed scintirenographic changes in acute rejection resemble those in ischemic injury [3]?

Methods

The most important data regarding the patients and the examinations are summarized in table 1. The diagnosis of acute rejection was based on clinical data and verified in most cases by renal angiography and biopsy. The severity of the rejection was judged from the maximal value of serum creatinine. In cases when dialysis treatment was needed the value of serum creatinine at the start of dialysis was used. The scintigrams and renograms were divided into seven groups (types a–g and 1–7, respectively) according to the degree of impairment of the accumulatory and excretory ability of the graft [3]. Regional renograms (cortex, medulla, pelvis) were constructed by a technique described in detail earlier [2, 3]. The uptake and excretory phases of the renograms representing the whole kidney and cortex were evaluated quantitatively according to a method described earlier [3]. The qualitative and quantitative evaluations performed in acute rejections were compared with those performed in ischemically damaged renal grafts [3].

Table 1. Data about the patients and the examinations

Immunosuppression: prednisolone and azathioprine	
Treatment of acute rejection: methylprednisolone i.v.	
Number of acute rejections	58
Rejections requiring dialysis treatment	28
Irreversible rejections	15
Test agent: ^{123}I-hippuran (Hoechst), dosage: 37 MBq	
Number of scintigrams	107
Number of renograms	92
Regional renography	77
Quantitative renography	34

Results

The typical scintigraphic findings during the development of acute rejection consisted of a decreased urinary output of hippuran causing a retention of the test agent in the graft. Simultaneously, the accumulatory ability of the graft decreased resulting in a low and heterogeneous renal accumulation of hippuran. During the restitution of the rejection the uptake was first improved and later the excretion.

Renography verified more objectively the above mentioned changes of the renal handling of hippuran in acute rejection. Furthermore, renography indicated a continuous but moderate delay of the time to the peak of the curve and the time to the start of the excretion to the urinary bladder with progressive impairment of the renogram (types 1–7).

Regional renography revealed that the cortical component in all types of the renogram constituted the main part (76–91%) of the total renogram (fig. 1). The shape of the total renogram was similar to that of the cortical curve. Thus, dysfunction of cortex was the cause of the observed deformations of the total renogram. When comparing findings of regional renography in acute rejection and ischemic damage [3], no significant differences were observed between these two conditions.

The relation between the different scintigraphic and renographic groups and the severity of the rejection is shown in figure 2a and b. A significant correlation ($p < 0.001$) between the two parameters was noticed. Scintigraphic and renographic changes of types e–g and 5–7 respectively appeared in severe rejection (serum creatinine > 500 μmol/l) mostly requiring dialysis treatment. In cases of scintigram and renogram of type g and 7 respectively the grafts were irreversibly damaged. Thus scintirenography gives a guideline about the prognosis of the renal damage caused by acute rejection.

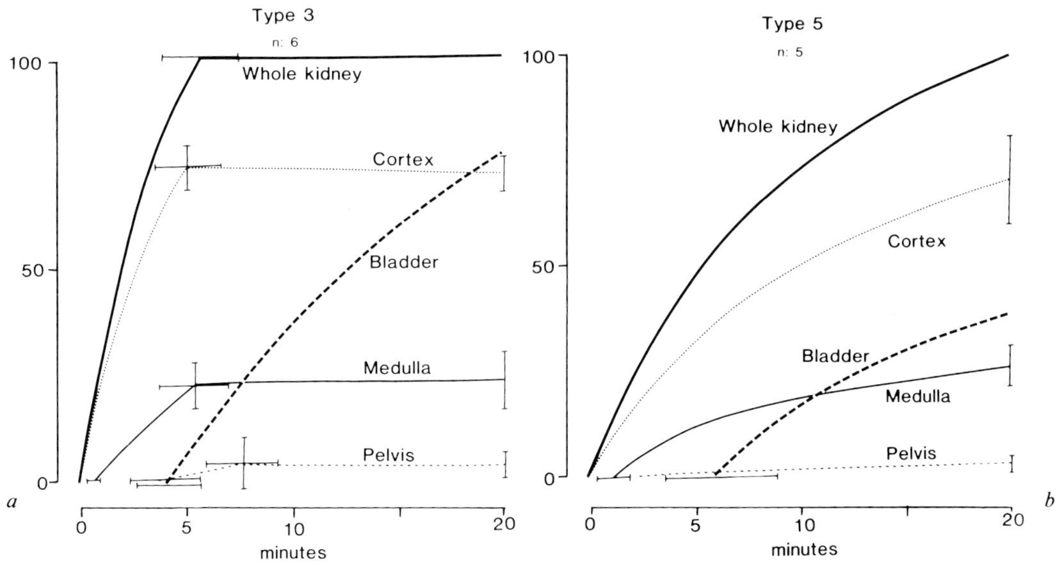

Fig. 1. Regional renography in the renographic groups of types 3 *(a)* and 5 *(b)*. The mean values (±1 SD) are indicated for different time intervals (time to curve onset and time to maximal amplitude) and for different amplitudes (amplitude at the maximum and at the end of the examination).

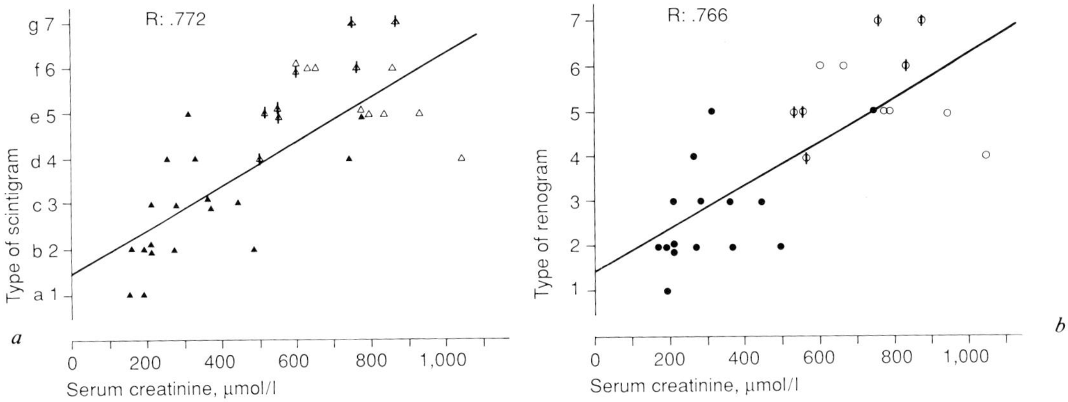

Fig. 2. The distribution of seven types of scintigrams *(a)* and renograms *(b)* (performed within ±3 days from day of maximal value of serum creatinine) in relation to the severity of the rejection according to the maximal value of serum creatinine. Unfilled circles and triangles indicate cases requiring dialysis treatment. Circles and triangles with vertical lines indicate irreversibly damaged grafts.

In the quantitative evaluation renograms of types 1–7 a gradual decrease of the accumulatory ability and a rapid fall of the excretory function of the whole graft as well as cortex were observed. The functional changes of the whole graft run parallel with those of cortex. A comparison between the quantitative parameters in acute rejection and those earlier published in ischemic damage [3] revealed no significant differences.

Conclusion

Acute rejection causes disturbed cortical kinetics of hippuran. The degree of the alteration is significantly correlated to the severity of the rejection. The intrarenal kinetic changes in acute rejection are qualitatively and quantitatively similar to those observed in ischemic damage. This fact supports the hypothesis that ischemia is an important cause of the altered renal handling of hippuran in acute rejection.

References

1 Lundgren G, Ekman L, Hansson E, et al: Renographic and autoradiographic studies during rejection in canine renal allografts. Acta Chir Scand 1967 (suppl 382).
2 Magnusson G, Elnäs S, Jansson, B, et al: Computer-controlled gamma-camera examination of human renal allografts using ^{123}I-hippuran. Findings in ischemic injury, acute rejection and urinary tract obstruction. Proc IVth Int Symp on Radionuclides in Nephrology, Boston 1978. Stuttgart, Thieme, 1980, pp 259–266.
3 Magnusson G, Groth C-G, Lewander, R, et al: Ischemic injury to renal allografts studied by gamma camera technique using ^{123}I-hippuran. Proc VIth Int Symp on Radionuclides in Nephrology, Lausanne 1986. Basel, Karger, 1987, pp 178–185.

G. Magnusson, MD, Department of Renal Medicine,
Huddinge University Hospital, S-141 86 Huddinge (Sweden)

Blaufox MD, Hollenberg NK, Raynaud C (eds): Radionuclides in Nephro-Urology. Contrib Nephrol. Basel, Karger, 1990, vol 79, pp 127–131

The Effects of Increased Dialysate Sodium Concentration on Skeletal Muscle and Subcutaneous Blood Flow during Hemodialysis

Dialysate Sodium and Regional Blood Flow

Mogens Hammer, Jens Kofoed-Johnsen

Department of Nephrology P 2132, Rigshospitalet, Copenhagen, Denmark

The frequency of hypotension and muscle pains during hemodialysis (HD) has been reported to be diminished by a high dialysate sodium concentration [1]. The present study was performed to study the effect of this HD technique on the peripheral circulation of skeletal muscles, and subcutaneous tissues.

Materials and Methods

Ten patients (2 females, 8 males, age 18–73 years) participated in the study. Diagnoses: glomerulonephritis (n = 6), pyelonephritis (n = 2), nephrosclerosis (n = 1), and reflux nephropathy (n = 1). None of the patients had been nephrectomized. All patients were treated with vitamins and phosphate binders.

The regular HD treatments were performed as 4–5 h of HD 3 times weekly (n = 8) or 6 h HD twice weekly (n = 2). HD were monitored and controlled by Gambro-Lundia^R AK-10 consoles with an ultrafiltration module (UFM), and a device enabling manual adjustments of dialysate conductance. The same type of dialyzer was used in both experiments: Proseries or GFseries (Gambro-Lundia^R, Sweden), depending on what the patient was accustomed to. The dialysate sodium concentration was either kept constant at 137 mEq/l, or altered from 147 mEq/l during the first 2 h of HD to 143 mEq/l during the third hour, and down to 137 mEq/l during the fourth hour.

Measurements of Cutaneous and Skeletal Muscle Blood Flows

Cutaneous and skeletal muscle blood flow changes were monitored by the ^{133}Xe washout technique, as previously described [2]. Skeletal muscle blood flow changes were measured in the anterior crural muscles, and cutaneous blood flow changes at an equal level on the opposite leg.

Gamma emission was measured by two cadmium-telluride (CdT) detectors (Novo Diagnostic Systems, Denmark) with time base of 30 s. The small detector size allowed that they could be fixed with double adhesive tape directly over the xenon depot. This technique yields a high counting efficiency and a constantcounting geometry without fixing the leg.

Gamma emission data were collected by a portable data retrieval system (Memolog 2a[R], Novo Diagnostic Systems). The data were transferred to a PC via a special Rs-232 interface (Novo Diagnostic Systems). Input, data analysis, and calculations of vascular resistances were performed with software developed by the authors.

Experimental Schedule

The doses of ^{133}Xe in 0.05 ml saline injected 1 h prior to HD were approximately 5×10^6 dps i.m. and 10^6 dps s.c. A period of at least 30 min was allowed to let the injection trauma vanish before measurements were started.

Arterial blood pressure (BPs) and heart rates (HRs) were measured, and blood flow and resistance calculated twice before and at least every 20 min during the first 2 h of HD, and every 30 min during the next 2 h by an automatic, printing sphygmomanometer. Central venous pressures were not measured but assumed to be constant, and 5 mm Hg.

Calculations of Blood Flows and Vascular Resistances

The washout of ^{133}Xe follows a monoexponential course [3, 4]. The fractional washout constant, k (min^{-1}), was calculated by the least squares method from the regression line of the logarithmically transformed counting rates. Calculations were automatically performed on 30 coordinate pairs, i.e. over a 15-min period, centered around times of BP measurements. If the regression coefficients were not significantly different from zero, blood flow was assigned a value of zero, and the resistance not calculated. The perfusion coefficients, f, was calculated from the following equation [5]: $f = k \times \lambda \times 100$ ($ml \times g^{-1} \times min^{-1}$), where λ (ml/g) is the tissue to blood partition coefficient, and k the xenon washout rate constant. The λ varies with the fat content of the tissue, but remains constant in a particular tissue during one series of experiments using the same depot of xenon [6]. As λ was assumed to remain constant, the relative blood flow was calculated as: $f_x/f_0 = k_x/k_0$, where k_o is the predialysis xenon washout rate constant. As the actual λ was unknown, the vascular resistance was calculated in arbitrary unit as: $R_x = \Delta P_x(A - V)/k_x \times 10^3$ ($mm\ Hg \times min \times 10^{-2}$), and was expressed as the relative resistance R_x/R_o [2].

Statistics

Significance of changes during HD were confirmed by the Kruskal-Wallis test, and a significance of intra- and interdialysis differences were tested by the Wilcoxon two-sample test. As limit of significance was used $p \leq 0.05$.

Results

Body Weight Reductions

Body weight (BW) reductions with constant and varying dialysate sodium concentrations were $3.2 \pm 0.5\%$ and $3.2 \pm 0.3\%$, respectively (mean ± SEM). Average BW decreased from 103 ± 1 to $99 \pm 1\%$ and from 104 ± 1 to $100 \pm 1\%$ of 'ideal weight', respectively.

Blood Pressure and Heart Rate

Average predialysis BPs and decrements were equal at the two occasions. Predialysis HRs were 76 ± 7 and $76 \pm 5\ min^{-1}$ (NS). After 4 h of HD with constant and varied dialysate sodium, HR was 86 ± 6 and $93 \pm 7\ min^{-1}$, respectively ($p < 0.02$).

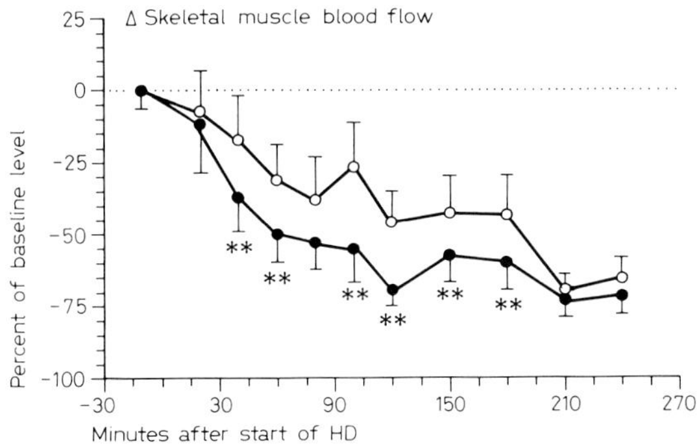

Fig. 1. Relative skeletal muscle blood flow in 10 patients during HD with either constant dialysate sodium (137 m*M*, ●) or initially high dialysate sodium (○). Blood flow decreased significantly with both techniques. During the initial 3 h, blood flow was significantly enhanced by high dialysate sodium (**$p < 0.05$). Means ± SEM.

Cutaneous Blood Flow and Resistance

Neither baseline cutaneous blood flows nor changes observed with the two techniques were significantly different. Neither did the changes of cutaneous vascular resistances differ significantly.

Skeletal Muscle Blood Flow and Vascular Resistance

The skeletal muscle blood flow decreased more slowly during the first hours of HD with high dialysate sodium, and remained at a higher level until the end of the dialysis (fig. 1). Skeletal muscle vascular resistance increased with varying dialysate sodium as well as with constant dialysate sodium. During the first 2 h of HD with constant sodium the increase was much more pronounced. However, due to great interindividual differences, the increase was not significantly different from that observed with varying dialysate sodium.

Subjective Symptoms and the Muscle Blood Flow

In patients who experienced muscle pains during HD, the subjective complaints were correlated to a significant decrease of the skeletal muscle blood flow. The relative blood flow changes were not greater in those patients who experienced muscle pains, but the blood flows were more oscillating. A high ultrafiltration (UF) rate generally caused a more rapid reduction of the skeletal muscle blood flow than that obtained with a lower UF rate, independent of the higher BW demanding the high UF rate. Figure 2 demonstrates the correlation between subjective symptoms and the

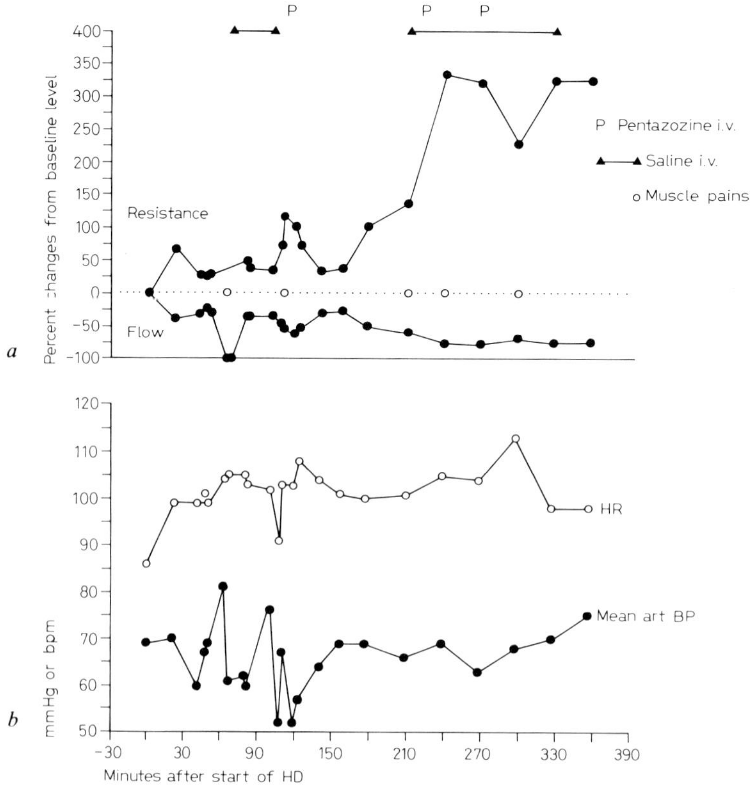

Fig. 2. *a* Correlation between muscle pain and relative skeletal muscle blood flow and resistance. *b* Concomitant changes of HR and mean arterial BP (diastolic BP + 1/3 pulse pressure).

changes of skeletal muscle blood flow, vascular resistance, HR, and mean BP in 1 patient during HD with constant dialysate sodium.

Discussion

The results of the present study suggest that a high dialysate sodium during the first hours of a HD session significantly diminishes the reduction of skeletal muscle blood flow induced by acetate buffered HD.

BP and HR changes as indicators of the status of the cardiovascular system are rather insensitive. From the observed BP and HR changes it is difficult to see a beneficial effect of an increased dialysate sodium. The results suggest that concomitant measurements of regional blood flow changes by the xenon washout technique is an appropriate way to evaluate different dialysis techniques. The placement of the detectors directly on skin surface over the muscle depot of xenon greatly enhanced the performance of this technique due to the higher counting efficiency, enabling measurements to be performed over several hours on the same depot [2]. The cardiac output was not measured in the present study. However, the greater HR and higher muscle blood flows suggest that a high dialysate sodium enhances the cardiac performance during HD.

The method used to vary the dialysate sodium concentration in the present study caused a parallel variation of the dialysate acetate concentration. The acetate ion has been suspected to be, at least in part, responsible for some of the cardiovascular side effects of HD [7, 8]. One might therefore speculate whether the beneficial effect of an increased dialysate sodium in the present study was partly obscured by the concomitant increase of dialysate acetate concentration.

References

1 Wehle B, Asaba H, Castenfors J, et al: The influence of dialysis fluid composition on the blood pressure response during dialysis. Clin Nephrol 1978;10:62–68.

2 Hammer M, Skagen K: Effects of small changes of plasma vasopressin on subcutaneous and skeletal muscle blood flow in man. Acta Physiol Scand 1986;127:67–73.

3 Larsen OA, Lassen NA, Quade F: Blood flow through human adipose tissue determined with radioactive xenon. Acta Physiol Scand 1966;66:337–345.

4 Lassen NA, Lindbjerg J, Munck O: Measurements of blood flow through skeletal muscle by intramuscular injection of xenon-133. Lancet 1964;i:686–689.

5 Kety SS: Theory and application of the exchange of inert gas at the lungs and tissues. Pharmacol Rev 1951;3:1–41.

6 Nielsen SL: Measurements of blood flow in adipose tissue from the washout of xenon-133 after atraumatic labeling. Acta Physiol Scand 1982;86:187–196.

7 Kirkendol PL, Devia CJ, Holbert RD: A comparison of the cardiovascular effects of sodium acetate, sodium bicarbonate and other potential sources of fixed base in hemodialysate solutions. Trans Am Soc Artif Intern Organs 1977;23:399.

8 Aizawa Y, Ohmori T, Imai K, et al: Depressant action of acetate upon the human cardiovascular system. Clin Nephrol 1977;8:477–481.

M. Hammer, MD, Department of Nephrology B 109, Herlev Hospital,
DK-2730 Herlev (Denmark)

Blaufox MD, Hollenberg NK, Raynaud C (eds): Radionuclides in Nephro-Urology. Contrib Nephrol. Basel, Karger, 1990, vol 79, pp 132–136

Assessment of Renal Volume in vivo Using SPECT

R. Wujanto, R.S. Lawson, H.J. Testa, R.A. Shields[1]

Department of Urology and Nuclear Medicine, Manchester Royal Infirmary, Manchester, UK

Advances in gamma camera and computer systems have enabled the use of a rotating gamma camera to acquire a set of radionuclide tomographic renal images using single photon emission computed tomography (SPECT). Apart from more detailed morphological examination of the kidneys, renal volume may be calculated in vivo from a set of transaxial images. The purpose of this paper is to evaluate the variation of renal volumes in patients with normal and scarred kidneys.

Materials and Methods

The gamma camera used in this study was an IGE 400A/T rotating gamma camera linked to an MDS A^3 computer system. SPECT studies were performed with the gamma camera set to acquire 64 images equally spaced around the patient. The images were therefore each separated by an arc of approximately 5.6 °. The acquisition time was 15 s/image, so each study took about 20 min to perform. The acquired data were stored in the computer on a 64 × 64 matrix. A set of transaxial images was reconstructed from the 64 planar views using the standard program supplied with the A^3 computer system. This utilised a filtered back projection algorithm employing a Butterworth filter with a cut off of 0.25 cycles per pixel and using opposing views to correct for attenuation. The reconstructed image in the computer is made up of small cubes, or voxels, which in this application measured $6 \times 6 \times 6\ mm^3$.

Renal volume was calculated using an in-house program by counting the total number of voxels in all the transaxial sections which exceeded a given threshold value. This threshold was specified as a percentage of the difference between the maximum count anywhere within the kidney and a background count outside the kidney. Previous study using kidney models showed that a threshold value of 37% would produce a result closest to the true volume [1].

Assessment of patients' renal volume in vivo was carried out on 56 consecutive patients who had been referred for radionuclide assessment of renal scarring. 1.5 MBq/kg body weight of ^{99m}Tc-DMSA was injected intravenously 3 h prior to gamma camera imaging. In addition

[1] We are very grateful to the Manchester and North West Kidney Research Association for funding this research project.

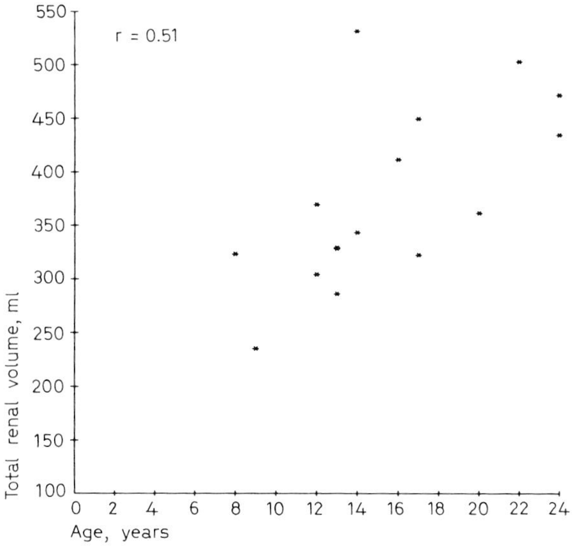

Fig. 1. Correlation between age and total renal volume.

to the traditional planar views, tomographic studies were performed and each renal volume was calculated as previously described using a threshold value of 37%. The detection of renal scarring was made primarily from the planar DMSA images. The results of renal volume for normal and scarred kidneys were compared. As the majority of patients also had a ^{123}I-hippuran renogram to assess dynamic renal function, the relative (split) renal function calculated from both the ^{123}I-hippuran study and the planar DMSA scan were compared with the calculated relative renal volume.

Results

Thirty-eight female and 18 male patients were studied. Their ages ranged from 6 to 70 years (mean 24.4 years). Three patients had solitary kidneys, therefore the study consisted of 109 kidneys from 56 patients. Scarring was demonstrable in 50 kidneys. Fifteen patients had bilateral scarring, 20 unilateral scarring and 18 normal kidneys bilaterally. The overall mean volume for the nonscarred kidneys was 205 ml (SD 56 ml) whereas that of the scarred kidneys was 143 ml (SD 74 ml) ($p < 0.001$). In the 18 patients with normal kidneys bilaterally, there was a weak but positive correlation between the total renal volume and the patients' age ($r = 0.51$) and body weight ($r = 0.68$) (fig. 1, 2). Good correlation was observed between the relative renal volume and the relative renal function

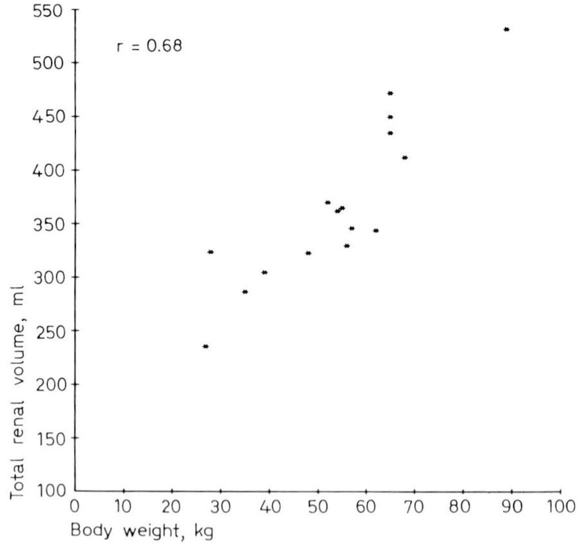

Fig. 2. Correlation between body weight and total renal volume.

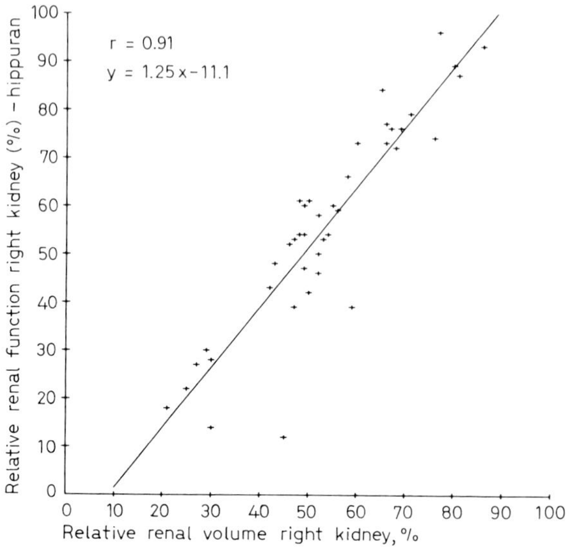

Fig. 3. Correlation of relative renal volume with relative renal function obtained from ^{123}I-hippuran study.

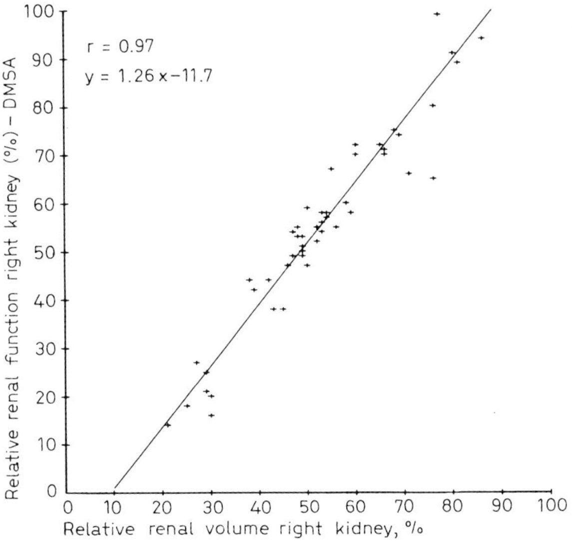

Fig. 4. Correlation of relative renal volume with relative renal function obtained from DMSA scan.

obtained from either the ^{123}I-hippuran study ($r = 0.91$) or the planar DMSA scan ($r = 0.97$) (figs. 3, 4). The mean volume of the 'normal' kidney, contralateral to a scarred kidney, was 226 ml in comparison with the mean volume of the kidneys from patients with two normal kidneys, which was 186 ml. Statistical analysis using the nonparametric Mann-Whitney U test showed that the difference was significant ($p = 0.005$). This finding strongly suggests that compensatory hypertrophy occurred in the 'normal' kidney contralateral to a scarred kidney.

Discussion

The application of SPECT to calculate patients' renal volume should be valuable in clinical practice. DMSA scanning is already considered to be one of the best methods of assessing renal scarring [2]. The additional SPECT study to measure renal volume does not require further injection of the radiopharmaceutical. It is recognised that the more severely scarred kidneys tend to be small and shrunken. Smellie et al. [3] attempted to classify the degree of scarring according to the appearance of the kidney from intravenous urography. While the criteria used for the classification have been widely accepted and adopted by the International Reflux Study Committee, this method lacks absolute quantification of renal volume. Our results showed that there was a wide variation in the measured volumes of both scarred and nonscarred kidneys, so a single measurement of renal volume is not so meaningful. However, serial measurement of functional renal volume should be useful in assessing the progress of renal scarring as well as the rate of growth of normal kidneys.

References

1 Wujanto R: The use of SPECT to calculate renal volume in vivo and its validation; MD thesis University of Manchester 1987, pp 97–117.

2 Merrick MV, Uttley WS, Wild SR: The detection of pyelonephritic scarring in children by radioisotope imaging. Br J Radiol 1980;53:544–556.

3 Smellie JM, Edwards D, Hunter N, et al: Vesico-ureteric reflux and renal scarring. Kidney Int 1975;8:S65–S72.

R. Wujanto, MD, FRCS, Department of Urology, Singapore General Hospital, Outram Road, Singapore 0316 (Singapore)

Blaufox MD, Hollenberg NK, Raynaud C (eds): Radionuclides in Nephro-Urology.
Contrib Nephrol. Basel, Karger, 1990, vol 79, pp 137–141

Long-Term Follow-Up of Separate Glomerular Filtration Rate in Partially Obstructed Kidneys

A. Piepsz[a, b], *H.R. Ham*[a], *M. Hall*[a], *M. Verboven*[b], *F. Collier*[c]

Departments of [a]Radioisotopes, [b]Pediatrics and [c]Pediatric Urology,
Free Universities of Brussels, Belgium

The aim of the present work was to evaluate the late effect of a nonoperated partial renal obstruction on separate glomerular filtration rate (SGFR), using two sets of data: (a) the first one is a long-term follow-up of SGFR in rats submitted to experimental partial ureteral obstruction; (b) the second one is a prospective study of asymptomatic neonates with pelviureteric junction (PUJ) obstruction detected prenatally.

Material and Methods

Experimental Rat Study

A left unilateral partial ureteric obstruction was created in 20 three-month-old male Wistar rats, using the technique described by Ulm and Miller [1] and repeated ^{99m}Tc-DTPA studies were performed. The animals were positioned on a small-field gamma camera and 2 mCi of ^{99m}Tc-DTPA were injected intravenously. A magnification of the images was obtained using the maximal zoom effect of the system. The data were recorded during 10 min, using 10 s frames. The radionuclide tests were performed before the creation of the obstruction, 15 days after the surgical procedure, and then approximately every 2 months, until the natural death of the animal.

The left to right clearance ratio was calculated using the mean slopes of the corrected ^{99m}Tc-DTPA renograms, between 40 and 70 s after intravenous injection. Since the aim of the study was to keep the rats alive as long as possible, no attempt was made to evaluate the absolute glomerular filtration of each kidney directly from the renal and the heart curve, in order to avoid the repeated blood sampling necessary for the calibration of the heart curve. Overall renal function was measured by counting, at the 10th minute after injection, the sum of both kidneys and bladder activity, which was expressed in percentage of the injected dose [2, 3]. Knowing the overall clearance and the left to right ratio, it became possible, by combining these two parameters, to obtain an estimation of the separate renal function. The whole kidney mean transit time was determined after deconvolution of the renographic curve by the heart curve. Two criteria of obstruction were taken into account: the demonstration of a persistent and important transit delay and the histological findings of enlargement of the cavities or dilatation of the collecting or convoluted tubules.

Prospective Study of Neonates

Fourteen neonates with prenatally detected unilateral PUJ stenosis were prospectively studied during a follow-up period of 1–6 years. The first ^{99m}Tc-DTPA test was performed around 1 month and was then regularly repeated. The SGFR was determined on the basis of the corrected renal curves and a calibrated heart curve, according to a previously published method [4]. For the furosemide test, we took into account the whole time activity curve as well as the postvoiding images. These 14 neonates were submitted to a similar protocol, based on the initial evaluation of SGFR. When SGFR was asymmetrical, the patients underwent a dismembered ureteropyeloplasty. One patient with symmetrical normal SGFR developed early severe signs of urinary tract infection and was therefore included in the surgical group. When SGFR was normal, a conservative attitude was adopted regardless of the results of the other radionuclide parameters.

Results

Experimental Rat Study

Before surgery, only small differences were observed between both kidneys, the ratio between the left and right kidney ranging between 0.78 and 1.09 (mean 0.94, SD 0.08). The SGFR results, expressed in percentage of the dose, were all included in a relatively small range of values (mean 19.6%, SD 0.9%). One month postoperatively, SGFR on the operated side was between 50 and 90% of the normal preoperative value. In 2 rats with accidental complete obstruction, the operated kidney was not visualized anymore. On the contralateral side, the mean postoperative value SGFR was 122% of the preoperative normal value, demonstrating variable functional compensation. After this first postoperative value, SGFR remained stable on the operated as well as on the contralateral side, until the natural death of the animal.

Prospective Study of Neonates

Separate Glomerular Filtration Rate. In the nonoperated patients, we observed, on the hydronephrotic as well as on the normal side, a progressive SGFR increase during the first year of life, due to the normal renal maturation. After the first year, SGFR remained stable within the normal range. In 1 patient, a sudden decrease of the renal function was observed around 1 year and the patient was therefore shifted in the surgical group. In the operated patients, the renal function on the hydronephrotic side generally remained below the normal range, sometimes after a slight increase of the function probably due to the maturation. On the contralateral side, SGFR was in the normal range without functional compensation.

Response to Furosemide. In the operated patients, we found generally no response to furosemide before surgery. After surgery a good or a partial response was always observed. In the nonoperated kidneys, the response to furosemide were variable from one test to another: sometimes we observed a complete kidney emptying; sometimes, in the same patient, only partial emptying occurred. In 1 patient, the furosemide test shifted from a partial response to no response at all. This was the patient who showed a sudden decrease of SGFR around 1 year of age and was operated upon thereafter.

Discussion

Two assumptions are regularly found in the strategy of management of pelviureteric junction stenosis. The first one is that nonoperated obstruction will progressively lead to the destruction of the kidney. This assumption is based on two sets of data: (a) The clinical and experimental observations on total obstructions, showing progressive irreversible destruction of the kidney. This model is however different from the partial obstruction existing in PUJ obstruction. (b) The immediate effect of an experimental partial obstruction, characterized by a rise of the pelvic pressure and, as a consequence, a decrease of SGFR.

The second assumption is that the surgical relief of the obstruction will improve the renal function. However, most of the studies are dealing with the improvement of the drainage function, demonstrated by the X-ray studies or by radionuclide techniques. Only few studies are quantifying the parenchymal function before and after surgery; it seems that if the preoperative function is altered, it will improve in a percentage of cases which is variable from one author to another.

Two long-term studies on patients with uropathies have been published [5, 6]. They are however retrospective studies, concerning heterogeneous groups of uropathies including mostly vesicoureteric reflux, urethral valves and bilateral obstruction with severe dysplasia and initial renal failure. It is for this reason that an experimental longitudinal long-term study was undertaken on partial ureteral obstruction in rats. The results of this study show that, at least in animals, after the initial postoperative period, the partial obstruction of the kidney does not produce further deterioration of the renal function and that the equilibrium is maintained throughout the life of the animal. It suggests that, in clinical routine, other criteria than only the fear of further degradation of the function should be taken into account when a surgical decision has to be considered.

This has led us to propose a prospective protocol in asymptomatic neonates with unilateral PUJ obstruction, mainly based on the initial value of SGFR: patients with low SGFR underwent a pyeloplasty with the hope to improve the renal function; patients with normal SGFR were not operated upon because, as far as we know, degradation of the parenchymal function in those patients has not been documented. In the nonoperated hydronephrotic kidneys, despite marked pelvic dilatation, SGFR generally remained normal and increased progressively, owing to the normal renal maturation. In 1 patient however, SGFR, after an initial rise, suddenly decreased; the absence of response to furosemide in this case could reflect a more severe obstruction and a sudden pressure rise, causing the decrease of parenchymal function. The absence of striking SGFR improvement in several operated cases is not surprising and has been the experience of many authors. This was certainly not related to secondary obstruction since the postoperative drainage function (furosemide test) markedly improved in all the cases. Owing to the present data, the initial protocol has now been modified: a conservative nonsurgical attitude is still recommended in cases with normal SGFR, as long as the furosemide test shows at least a partial response; on the basis of one case, we consider that an absence of response to furosemide on successive tests (including postvoiding images) after the age of 6 months might represent a supplementary risk of renal function damage and the patient will probably be referred for surgery. It is obvious that this protocol, based on radionuclide parameters, must only be considered as a guideline, owing to the small number of cases included in the study and the need for further validation of the modified protocol. Moreover, this protocol should be modulated by the appearance at any moment of clinical symptoms or by a sudden increase of the grade of hydronephrosis on ultrasound.

This experimental study was undertaken in order to evaluate on a long-term basis the progression of the SGFR in a series of young rats submitted to a partial obstruction of the left ureter. We observed, like other authors, an initial variable postoperative SGFR decrease, depending on the degree of provoked obstruction. However, after this initial period, SGFR remained stable until the natural death of the animal.

The second study was a clinical prospective study on 14 asymptomatic neonates with PUJ obstruction detected on prenatal ultrasound. When SGFR was abnormal, with very asymmetrical left and right function, the patients underwent a pyeloplasty, with the hope to improve the renal function. When SGFR was normal, a conservative attitude was chosen, no matter the results of the furosemide test. In the operated patients, despite a slight SGFR increase, probably related to the normal renal maturation during the first year of life, SGFR generally remained below the normal range. In the nonoperated hydronephrotic kidneys with initial normal function, SGFR constantly remained in the normal range, during a follow-up period of 1–6 years. In only 1 patient, we observed a significant SGFR decrease after 1 year and the patient was shifted into the surgical group. This patient was precisely the only one with a persistent nonresponse to furosemide. It was therefore decided to modify slightly the protocol and to operate the patients with a persistent absence of response to furosemide after the age of 6 months. This protocol should be constantly modulated by the appearance of clinical symptoms or by a sudden increase of hydronephrosis on ultrasound.

References

1 Ulm AH, Miller F: An operation to produce experimental reversible hydronephrosis in dogs. J Urol 1962;88:337–341.
2 Lee TY, Constable AR, Cranage RW: A method for GFR determination without blood samples in routine renal scintigraphy with ^{99m}Tc-DTPA; in Tauxe (ed): Radionuclides in Nephrology. London, Academic Press, 1982, pp 197–202.
3 Piepsz A, Froideville JL, Kinthaert J, et al: Reproducibility of three methods of renal clearance estimation without blood samples by means of ^{99m}Tc-DTPA; in Blaufox (ed): Radionuclides in Nephrology. Basel, Karger 1987, pp. 77–81.
4 Piepsz A, Dobbeleir A, Erbsmann F: Measurement of separate kidney clearance by means of ^{99m}Tc-DTPA complex and a scintillation camera. Eur J Nucl Med 1977;2:173–177.
5 Mayor G, Genton N, Torrado A, et al: Renal function in obstructive nephropathy: long-term effect of reconstructive surgery. Pediatrics 1975;56:740–747.
6 Warshaw BL, Edelbrock HH, Ettenger RB, et al: Progression to end-stage renal disease in children with obstructive uropathy. J Pediat 1982;100:183–187.

A. Piepsz, Department of Radioisotopes, Hôpital Saint-Pierre, 322 rue Haute, B–1000 Brussels (Belgium)

Blaufox MD, Hollenberg NK, Raynaud C (eds): Radionuclides in Nephro-Urology.
Contrib Nephrol. Basel, Karger, 1990, vol 79, pp 142–146

Development of Renal Scars after Acute Nephronia in Childhood: A Study of Sequential DMSA Scans

I.G. Verber, S.T. Meller

Queen Mary's Hospital for Children, Carshalton, and The Royal Marsden Hospital, Sutton, Surrey, UK

Renal scarring often follows renal involvement (acute nephronia) during urinary tract infection in young children and DMSA scans are the most sensitive imaging method for detecting such involvement [1]. Renal scarring is the main determinant of outcome following childhood urinary tract infection [2]. Although vesico-ureteric reflux is important because of its well-described association with scarring [3], there is no evidence that reflux alone is harmful. However, it is not known how often kidneys with acute changes will be permanently damaged nor how much damage is sustained at the first infection and how much is the result of repeated insults. Serial studies of kidneys using excretory urography have been published [4] but here the appearance of new defects may be due to contraction of original scars by fibrosis so it is uncertain whether kidneys unscarred at first infection are subsequently at risk. We report the follow-up DMSA scans on 45 children who were first scanned within a month of a first urinary tract infection.

Patients and Methods

Over a 3-year period (1982–1984), 115 children under the age of 5 years presented with a first symptomatic urinary tract infection (UTI), proven by urinary culture. A DMSA scan (CIS UK Ltd) was performed as part of an investigation protocol which also included micturating cysto-urethrography. The methodology and the results have been reported previously [1]. Forty-five children have subsequently been rescanned and their results form this present study. The mean age at time of the first scan was 2.04 years with a range of 12 days to 4.9 years and at time of the second scan 4.29 years with a range of 33 weeks to 9.5 years. The interval between scans was a mean of 2.25 years with a range of 25 weeks to 6.3 years.

All children with reflux received continuous prophylactic antibiotics in the period between the 2 DMSA scans or, in 17 cases where reflux was corrected surgically, until 6 months after operation. The DMSA scan results were reviewed without knowledge of other imaging results or clinical course. Each kidney was classified as being abnormal (i.e. showing a definite cortical defect or having diffuse abnormality of DMSA uptake) or as being normal. The kidneys on the second scan were additionally classified as deteriorated, unchanged or improved as compared to the first scan. Relative percentage uptake of DMSA had been calculated by region of interest analysis in 89 of the 90 scans reviewed.

Results

There were 49 kidneys initially having defects of which 31 had reflux. Forty (80%) of them still had defects present at follow-up including 12 kidney units without reflux. There was no relationship between changes in the appearance of the kidneys on the DMSA scans and the presence or degree of reflux at presentation. The remaining 9 kidneys had no defects at follow-up. Resolution of defects was not related to the time interval between scans.

Forty-one kidneys were initially normal; 18 had reflux but 9 of these were subsequently surgically corrected, thus 32 kidneys had no reflux during the study period. Seven of these were exposed to breakthrough infection. Three kidneys had uncorrected reflux (two grade 2 and one grade 3) but no breakthrough infections. None of these 35 kidneys developed defects. Six kidneys had breakthrough infections in the presence of reflux – three grade 1 and three grade 3. Two of these latter kidneys (in the same child) developed widespread defects.

There was no correlation between changes in appearance between the two scans and the presence of reflux alone or the occurrence of breakthrough infection alone, but kidneys with grade 3 reflux *and* breakthrough infection had a greater risk of showing deterioration, 3 out of 8 cases, than those without this combination, 3 out of 82 cases ($p = 0.001$ Fisher exact test two-tailed).

Where one kidney was normal it was reasonable to assume that any reduction in relative DMSA uptake by an affected contralateral kidney indicated an absolute loss of function. There were 30 children with unilateral abnormalities in whom divided DMSA uptake was measured. There was a very close relationship between DMSA uptake in kidneys at the first and at the second scan (fig. 1) and this applied equally to those kidneys with or without reflux or breakthrough indicating that the damage sustained at the first infection is the main determinant of functional outcome. There was a significant difference between the initial uptake of DMSA between those kidneys where cortical defects subsequently improved (43.1% (SD 5.5)) and those which showed no improvement (34.7% (SD 12.2) $p < 0.02$, Student's t test). No kidney with an uptake of less than 35% showed any improvement of associated cortical defects (fig. 2).

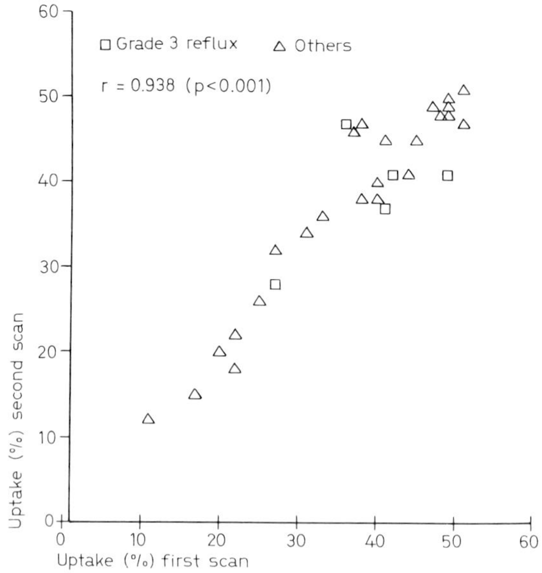

Fig. 1. Relationship between DMSA uptake (%) at first and second scan in unilaterally scarred kidneys.

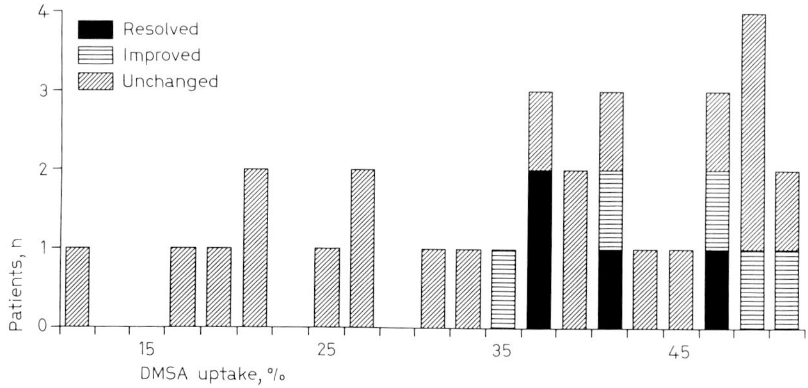

Fig. 2. Outcome of renal defects related to initial DMSA uptake (%) in unilaterally scarred kidneys.

Discussion

When cortical defects are present on an initial DMSA scan there is a high risk of permanent renal damage. It has been suggested that some defects seen on scans performed within 3 months of a urinary tract infection may be transient [5] and this has led to the idea that scans should not be performed within this period [6]. We have shown that 80% of these changes persisted. We believe waiting for 3 months before performing these scans is undesirable as it will result in delay in identifying children with kidneys at risk.

The defects that do not persist probably represent an acute nephronia which resolves; recent animal work has shown that kidneys with defects on DMSA scan always have a corresponding pathological lesion [7]. Kidneys which are undamaged after a first infection can occasionally develop significant scarring at subsequent infection [4], but this is a rare event and in our series was only seen in 1 child who had bilateral grade 3 reflux. The reason why we found so few new scars might be because DMSA scans are more sensitive in detecting initial parenchymal changes than intravenous urography on which previously reported studies have depended [8].

Most renal defects remained unchanged regardless of features on presentation or subsequent clinical course. This suggests that for most children the initial infection is the cause of damage and subsequent breakthrough infection makes little difference. It has been suggested that those kidneys with compound renal papillae, making them more susceptible to damage, are all affected by the first infection – the so-called 'big-bang' theory [9] and our findings would support this.

An interesting feature of our original cohort [1] was the high incidence of defects in the absence of reflux and 12 of these have now been shown to be permanent suggesting at least 18% of permanent renal defects develop in the absence of reflux compared with 2% previously reported in a study where intravenous urography was accepted as the standard [10].

We have examined the outcome of kidneys in relation to the initial investigations: the presence of reflux predicts an abnormal outcome with a sensitivity of 0.68 and a specificity of 0.58; grade 3 reflux has a sensitivity of 0.45 and a specificity of 0.9 and an abnormal DMSA scan within a month of the first infection has a sensitivity of 0.95 and a specificity of 0.81.

DMSA scans have led to a clearer understanding of the factors which determine the development of chronic pyelonephritis and we believe that they are an essential modality in the investigation of urinary tract infection in the under five age group.

References

1 Verber IG, Strudley MR, Meller ST: ^{99m}Tc dimercaptosuccinic acid (DMSA) scan as first investigation of urinary tract infection. Arch Dis Child 1988;63:1320–1325.
2 Sacks SH, Verrier-Jones K, Roberts R, et al: Effect of symptomless bacteruria in childhood on subsequent pregnancy. Lancet 1987;ii:991–994.
3 Scott JES, Stansfeld JM: Ureteric reflux and kidney scarring in children. Arch Dis Child 1968;43:468–470.
4 Filly R, Friedland GW, Govan DE, et al: Development and progression of clubbing and scarring in children with recurrent urinary tract infections. Radiology 1974;113:145–153.
5 Merrick MV, Uttley WS, Wild SR: The detection of pyelonephritic scarring in children by radio-isotope imaging. Br J Radiol 1980;53:544–556.
6 Thelle T, Biskjaer N: Combined (^{99m}Tc) DMSA kidney scintigraphy and (^{131}I) hippuran renography in children with urinary tract infections. Acta Paediatr Scand 1985;74:720–725.
7 Parkhouse HF, Godley ML, Cooper J, et al: Renal imaging with ^{99m}Tc-DMSA in the detection of acute pyelonephritis; an experimental study in the pig. Nucl Med Commun 1989;10:63–79.
8 Smellie JM, Ransley PG, Normand ICS, et al: Development of new renal scars – a collaborative study. Br Med J 1985;290:1957–1960.
9 Ransley PG, Risdon RA: Papillary morphology in infants and young children. Urol Res 1975;3:111–113.
10 Shah KJ, Robins DG, White RHR: Renal scarring and vesico-ureteric reflux. Arch Dis Child 1978;53:210–217.

S.T. Meller, FRCP, Children's Department, Royal Marsden Hospital,
Sutton, Surrey SM2 5PT (UK)

Blaufox MD, Hollenberg NK, Raynaud C (eds): Radionuclides in Nephro-Urology.
Contrib Nephrol. Basel, Karger, 1990, vol 79, pp 147–155

Correlation between Scintigraphic Lesions and Renal Scarring in Intravenous Urogram in Children with Normal Relative Uptake of DMSA and Evaluation of Normal Kidney Findings of DMSA Scan

A. Piepsz, T. Tamminen-Möbius

For International Reflux Study in Children, DMSA Working Group[1]

^{99m}Tc-DMSA is an excellent marker of any functioning renal tissue [1]. We have used DMSA uptake ratio for long-term follow-up of 402 children with moderate to severe vesicoureteral reflux (VUR). In most of the children, DMSA scintigrams were made concomitantly with the uptake test. 67% of these children had lesions of kidney parenchyma in intravenous urogram (IVU) and 72% of these lesions fulfilled the criteria of renal scar, i.e. they had areas of thin parenchyma with distorted calyx. It has been suggested recently by several authors [2, 4] that DMSA scintigram should be the first-choice investigation in children with VUR instead of IVU. Others think that DMSA scan is good as a complementary investigation only [5, 6]. We found the interpretation of DMSA scintigram in a randomly selected group of 40 children (out of our 402 children) problematic [5]. Agreement about normality/abnormality between three independent observers was only reached in 35% of children. Therefore, we considered it essential to evaluate DMSA scintigram findings more detailed. Which kind of defects were observed and is it possible to define them? How often are they found in scarred and unscarred kidneys with or without VUR but without recent urinary tract infection?

[1] Paper given by A. Piepsz and drafted by Tytti Tamminen-Möbius (Coordinator). Other DMSA Working Group Members: G. Fueger, A. Kivisaari, Ch. Reiners. Participating Hospitals and the Principal Investigators: University Children's Hospital, Bonn, FRG: Rudolf Mallmann. University Children's Hospital, Universite Libre de Bruxelles, Belgium: Michelle Hall. University Children's Hospital, Essen, FRG (Coordinating Center): Hermann Olbing (Chairman). University Children's Hospital, Gothenburg, Sweden: Ulf Jodal. Department of Urology, University of Hamburg, FRG: Rainer Busch. University Children's Hospital, Helsinki, Finland: Olli Koskimies. University Children's Hospital, Oulu, Finland: Juhani Seppänen. Karolinska Institutet, St. Göran's and Sachska Children's Hospitals, Stockholm, Sweden: Anita Aperia.

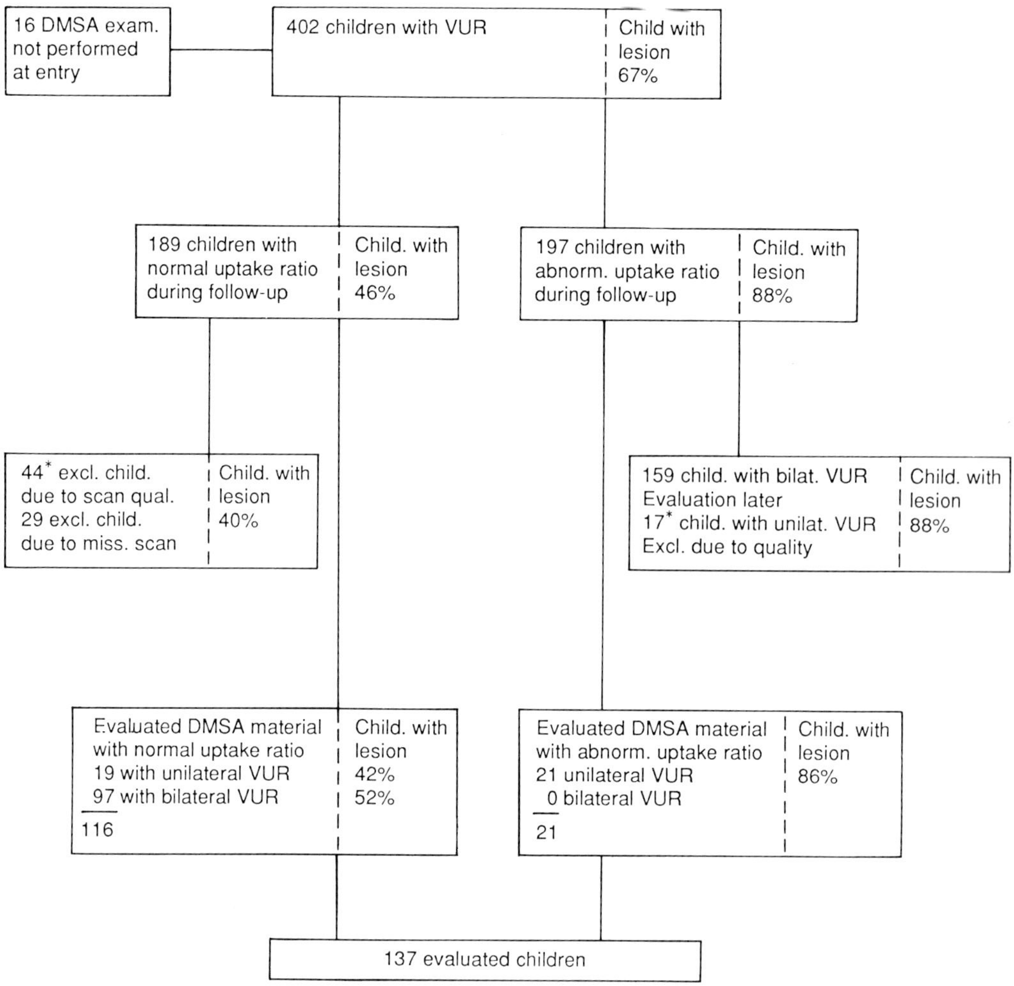

*61 children all from one hospital with digitalized scans with an unacceptable coloured scale.

Fig. 1. DMSA examinations of the International Reflux Study in Children.

Patients

116 patients (19 with unilateral VUR and 97 with bilateral VUR) having normal uptake ratio of DMSA and 21 additional children having abnormal DMSA ratio with unilateral VUR were included (fig. 1). At entry to the study, all these children had a VUR which distended upper urinary tract (international grades III or IV) in bilateral cases at least on one side. 69 children had 98 kidneys with VUR at the time of the comparison between IVU and DMSA. No child had urinary tract infection at the time of this comparison.

73 patients with normal uptake ratio could not be analyzed because of image quality (44 cases) or because of missing scans (29 cases). 197 patients with abnormal DMSA ratio were left out of the analysis (88% of these children had parenchymal lesions), except the 21 out of 38 children with unilateral VUR having an acceptable scan and abnormal DMSA ratio.

Each child has been followed for at least 3 years. An IVU was performed together with DMSA scan at entry and after a follow-up of 6, 18 and 54 months. To minimize the cumulative radiation in these children, all radiological investigations were performed with lowest possible radiation dose.

Methods

^{99m}Tc-DMSA was injected intravenously (approx. 0.74 MBq/kg body weight) and the relative activity in the kidney region was measured 3–4 h after injection in a supine-positioned patient with a gamma camera underneath the table. Simultaneously, an image with 300,000 counts was made on Polaroid or X-ray film. When such an analogue image was not available, special computer handling was used to produce a comparable image. Only scans with visible pelviocalyceal system were considered acceptable for analysis.

IVU were performed with a bolus injection of 50 or 60% triiodinated agents (4 ml/kg body weight in newborns and 2 ml/kg body weight in older children). Exposures were taken immediately after injection, at 5 and 10 min. Careful patient preparation before IVU was strongly attributed. Visualization of total kidney outline and pelviocalyceal system were the criteria for good quality IVU and only such an IVU was acceptable for comparison with good quality DMSA scans.

Each patient was examined several times over 3–5 years with both methods and all available examinations were evaluated longitudinally, DMSA scans and IVU pictures totally independently from each other, by at least two 'blind' observers (also the presence of VUR was not known to the observers). Any discrepancies in the analysis of IVU or DMSA pictures were solved in sessions with 2–5 investigators separately for IVU and DMSA. One pair of the examinations (IVU/DMSA) in each child was chosen by the Study Coordinator for comparison based on the quality and timing of these examinations. In 21 children the comparison was made at entry to the study and in 59 children after 18 months of follow-up and in 57 children, the latest examinations, 54 months after entry, were compared with IVU.

The kidney outlines and pelves in IVU were double traced by two independent observers. In each child several IVUs were available for the detection of the morphological lesions of reflux nephropathy and therefore, IVU was considered to be an adequate standard method for specificity and sensitivity analysis of DMSA scan in finding morphological lesions. Because reflux may cause functional or vascular changes in kidney parenchyma not detectable by IVU, additional analysis of specificity and sensitivity of DMSA scan was performed in children with unilateral reflux having normal contralateral kidney.

The following categories of abnormalities in DMSA scan were first worked out in a group of 52 children with DMSA uptake ratio within 50 ± 5%. Twelve main categories were seen:

(1) Flattened or concave kidney outline with adjacent hypoactive tissue.

(2) Concave kidney outline adjacent to normally active tissue.

(3) Inactive area, the hole surrounded by functional tissue. (Such holes are frequently seen centrally in upper and/or lower poles of kidneys, and are a normal finding in these typical locations.)

(4) Flattened kidney outline without adjacent hypoactive area. (Flattened outline with adjacent hyperactive tissue is considered to be a normal finding and frequently seen in upper lateral part of left kidney, where the spleen flattens the kidney outline.)

(5) Deformed kidney outline with or without local defect or small kidney with local defects.

(6) Shortening of kidney vertical axis, rounded kidney without local defects.

(7) Shortening of kidney horizontal axis in upper or lower pole, pear-shapped kidneys without local defects.

(8) Shortening of kidney horizontal axis, slender kidney without local defects (exception: slender kidney with a hyperactive lateral margin is a normal, but rotated kidney).

(9) Hypoactivity of whole upper and/or lower pole with normal kidney outline.

(10) Multiple small hypoactive areas with normal kidney shape (marginal notching defects).

(11) Small normal-looking kidney without local defects.

(12) Prominent concavity of kidney hilar area. This type of abnormality may be seen together with all the other forms of DMSA defects given above. It is a sign of dilated kidney pelvis and not a parenchymal lesion. This category will be analyzed separately later on and the findings are not included in this paper.

The parenchymal lesion in IVU were defined as follows:

(1) Major lesions: parenchymal thinning with distorted calyx, kidney scars.

(2) Minor lesions: parenchymal thinning without calyceal deformity, arrested 'parenchymal lesion'. The minimal thickness of parenchyma was measured in upper pole, midzone and lower pole and compared with the normogram of normal children [7].

Results

DMSA scan showed correctly 32/34 normal kidneys without VUR. Overall specificity in finding radiologically normal kidneys was 0.79 (table 1) with a sensitivity of 0.87 for major lesions and 0.71 for minor lesions in 137 evaluated children. The sensitivity of DMSA scan in children with normal uptake ratio was 0.78 overall, 0.71 for minor lesions and 0.83 for major lesions, with a specificity of 0.74. Thus, inclusion of 21 children with unilateral reflux, but abnormal uptake ratio in the analyzed material, had only a minor influence on these values.

The suggested categories of DMSA lesions were seen very variably within corresponding radiological lesions (table 2). A contour abnormality without adjacent hypoactive tissue predicted a kidney region with minor or

Table 1. DMSA scintigram findings compared with IVU in 274 kidneys of 137 children with or without VUR (any time in past or present)

IVU findings	DMSA findings					
	norm. scan	local defects[1]	deformed kidney	small kidney	abnorm. kidney shape	total
No lesion						
VUR –	32	2	0	0	0	34
VUR +	98	36	0	2	2	138
Minor lesion						
VUR –	4	0	0	0	1	5
VUR +	8	21	4	1	2	36
Major lesion						
VUR –	0	1	0	0	0	1
VUR +	8	18	27	4	3	60
	150	78	31	7	8	274

Sensitivity: overall 0.80, for major lesion 0.87, for minor lesions 0.71.
Specificity: overall 0.76, for kidneys with nonexistent VUR 0.94.
[1] Six kidneys with hypoactivity in one of the kidney poles and three with marginal notching defects included.

major lesion only in 37% of cases whereas similar contour abnormality with a defect was successful in finding lesions in 57% of the cases. The opposite, hypoactive tissue without contour deformity was very seldom a sign of morphological kidney lesion. A vascular pathogenicity is a likely cause for such defects in DMSA scan (frequently seen with acute pyelonephritis). As expected, a hole in DMSA scan (PA view) cannot very reliably predict a parenchymal lesion. A pear-shaped kidney was considered to have a defect in upper or lower pole and in the midzone, but mostly (10/16) this was not the case. Small normal-looking kidneys in DMSA scan were generally small also in IVU. However, 12/21 of the small normal-looking kidneys had parenchymal lesions in IVU. There were altogether 533 kidney regions without a lesion according to both methods out of 587 radiologically normal kidney areas, again showing the high specificity of DMSA scan.

We also tested the overall sensitivity and specificity of DMSA scan separately in all 40 children with unilateral VUR. The values were close to 85% both for specificity and sensitivity confirming that the criteria used for

Table 2. DMSA lesion categories and their localization in comparison with lesions seen in IVU

IVU findings	DMSA normal	Local DMSA defects in categories				General DMSA lesions in categories				
	0	1	2	3	4	5	6/7/8	9	10	11
Upper Pole										
No lesion	146	13	2	6	3	1	1	5	2	2
Minor	14	9	4	2	3	3	3	1	0	1
Major	7	9	2	2	0	27	1	0	1	4
Total	167	31	8	10	6	31	5	6	3	7
Midzone										
No lesion	210	2	4	0	2	2	7	0	2	4
Minor	7	0	0	1	0	1	0	0	0	3
Major	9	1	2	1	0	14	1	0	1	0
Total	226	3	6	2	2	17	8	0	3	7
Lower Pole										
No lesion	177	7	6	1	6	3	2	3	2	3
Minor	13	4	0	0	0	6	0	0	0	2
Major	4	6	0	1	2	22	1	0	1	2
Total	194	17	6	2	8	31	3	3	3	7
Total	587	51	20	14	16	79	16	9	9	21
Predictive values	0.91	0.57	0.40	0.50	0.31	0.92	0.38	0.11	0.33	0.57

detecting lesions were in general correctly chosen even if the predictability of a lesion and its exact localization in IVU with some types of DMSA findings was low. If one would consider that all the DMSA findings in categories with positive predictability less than 50% were normal, the overall sensitivity of DMSA scan would have been for major lesions 0.75 and for minor lesions 0.46, with a specificity of 0.90.

In 62% of children, IVU and DMSA were in agreement and there was no difference in children with unilateral or bilateral VUR. 8% of children would have passed with normal DMSA scan, although they had lesions in IVU (nine times in one kidney and twice in both kidneys). DMSA scan underestimated kidney lesions only in 4% of the children and overestimated them in 26% of the cases (table 3).

Table 3. DMSA scintigram findings compared with IVU in 137 children with VUR (any time in past or at present)

Finding in IVU	DMSA scintigram findings					Children, n
	both kidneys normal	one kidney normal, other with			both kidneys abnorm.	
		local defects	deformed or small	shape abnorm.		
Both kidneys normal	32	17	2	4	6	61
One kidney abnormal	9	20	12	3	6	50
Both kidneys abnormal	2	3	2	1	18	26
Total	43	40	16	8	30	137

Discussion

The classical appearance of a pyelonephritic scar with indentation of renal outline overlying clubbed calyx is an end stage of such a lesion. It has been thought that all scars would progress to their end stage, but the experience of the International Reflux Study in Children does not support such a view. We have seen frequently scars with thinned parenchyme and distorted calyx without indentation of kidney outline and clubbing of calyx. In most of our children, no progress of the scars has been observed. We have also seen many minor parenchymal lesions which might or might not progress into a scar. Identification of such minor lesions is clinically very important because of their potential risk of further scarring [8]. Therefore, one aim of this study was to test how accurately such minor kidney lesions can be detected with DMSA scans; the main aim being the evaluation of the criteria for normal and abnormal DMSA scan.

83% of scarred kidneys were found with DMSA scan even in the group of children having a normal DMSA uptake ratio. 87% of kidneys with deformed kidney outline in DMSA scan (cat. 5) had major lesions in urogram and none of these kidneys was normal. 47% of kidneys with local defects in DMSA had no corresponding morphological lesion in intravenous urogram, 28% had minor lesions and only 25% major lesions. How should these findings be interpreted? It is possible that morphologically normal kidneys do have lesions of more functional character which are detectable only with DMSA scan as has been suggested by others [2–4]. The significance of such lesions can be tested together with the observed growth of these kidneys later on. It is well known that parenchymal lesions are often associated with poor kidney growth and it may be that the discrepant lesions seen only in DMSA scan would also affect kidney growth. On the other hand, the persistence of VUR may also cause functional lesions of kidney parenchyma. This will be evaluated by a longitudinal analysis of out data later on.

50% of scintigram findings were not agreed to be normal or abnormal by all of our investigators. The analysis of DMSA was greatly affected by the quality of DMSA scan (excellent quality even increased discrepant opinions). Exact definitions of local and general lesions in DMSA scans helped in finding an agreement. Flattening of contour with hyperactive tissue adjacent to this was agreed to be a normal finding and indeed, only 1/15 such areas had a scar. Centrally located symmetrical holes were also considered as normal variations in posterior/anterior views. An oblique view could have been helpful in differentiating such holes either as parenchymal defects or as dilated calyces with normal parenchyma. Obviously, because of lacking information about calyces, the decision of normal kidney with abnormal shape cannot be made with DMSA scintigram.

In conclusion, we can say that DMSA is an excellent marker of renal tissue with high specificity and good sensitivity, even in children with normal DMSA uptake ratio. In order to be able to find minor lesions, e.g. thinning of parenchyma, scans have to be analyzed very thoroughly. Our definitions of defects helped in describing the abnormalities of DMSA. The defined types of DMSA defects had variable predictive values for lesions in IVU of the corresponding kidney region, suggesting a secondary nature of DMSA defects. We were pleased to see that 88% of the children with abnormal DMSA uptake ratio had a lesion at least in one of the kidneys.

References

1 Gordon I: Indications for technetium-99m-dimercaptosuccinic acid scan in children. J Urol 1987;137:464–467.

2 Goldraich NP, Ramos OL, Goldraich IH: Urography versus DMSA scan in children with vesicoureteric reflux. Pediatr Nephrol 1989;3:1–5.

3 Verber IG, Strudley MR, Meller ST: ^{99m}Tc-dimercaptosuccinic acid (DMSA) scan as first investigation of urinary tract infection. Arch Dis Child 1988;63:1320–1325.

4 Stoller ML, Kogan BA: Sensitivity of technetium-99m-dimercaptosuccinic acid for the diagnosis of chronic pyelonephritis: Clinical and theoretical considerations. J Urol 1986;135: 977–980.

5 Tamminen-Möbius T, Olbing H: ^{99m}Tc-DMSA uptake – percentage test and scintigram as a method for evaluation of kidney parenchyme defects in children with vesico-ureteral reflux; in Murakami K, Kitagawa T, Yabuta K, et al (eds): Recent Advances in Pediatric Nephrology. Proc Seventh Int Congr of Pediatric Nephrology, Tokyo, Amsterdam, Excerpta Medica, 1987.

6 Smellie JM: The DMSA scan and intravenous urography in the detection of renal scarring. Pediatr Nephrol 1989;3:6–8.
7 Claesson I, Jacobsson B, Olsson T, et al: Assessment of renal parenchymal thickness in normal children. Acta Radiol (Diagn) 1981;22:305–316.
8 Tamminen-Möbius T, Olbing H, Bachmann HJ: The development of segmental scarring in previously normal kidneys seen in three children with vesicoureteric reflux. Klin Pädiat 1982;194:137–139.

Tytti Tamminen-Möbius, MD, International Reflux Study in Children,
Coordination Center, University Children's Hospital, Hufelandstrasse 55,
D–4300 Essen 1 (FRG)

Blaufox MD, Hollenberg NK, Raynaud C (eds): Radionuclides in Nephro-Urology.
Contrib Nephrol. Basel, Karger, 1990, vol 79, pp 156–160

Comparison of Conventional Furosemide Diuresis Renography with Direct Intrapelvic Infusion Renography

Kazuo Itoh[a], *Kotarou Taniguchi*[b], *Masami Nantani*[b], *Katsuya Nonomura*[b], *Masayori Furudate*[a], *Tomohiko Koyanagi*[b]

Departments of [a]Nuclear Medicine and [b]Urology, Hokkaido University School of Medicine, Sapporo, Japan

Furosemide-augmented diuresis renography has been proposed as an effective means to distinguish nonobstructed dilatation of the upper urinary system from significant mechanical obstruction [7, 9]. The method is simple and noninvasive. However, we encountered several false-positive cases which showed completely obstructed curves by conventional diuretic renography and the absence of the obstruction by subsequently performed Whitaker test.

Materials and Methods

Fifteen patients (13 male, 2 female; age range 2–66 years) with percutaneous antegrade pelvicalyceal nephrostomy for the treatment of hydronephrosis and renal stones provided 16 renal units for study. Hydronephrosis was due to pelviureteric junction stenosis in 10 patients, megaureter in 1, retrocaval ureter in 1, renal stone in 1 and malignant stricture caused by invasion of uterine cervical cancer in 1.

All of the patients were asked to drink an additional 300 ml of water to make them normally hydrated 15–20 min prior to the conventional diuretic renography. ^{99m}Tc-diethylenetriaminepentaacetic acid (^{99m}Tc-DTPA) at a dose of 4 MBq/kg (with a maximal dose of 296 MBq) was administered intravenously keeping the patient in a supine position. Standard renal scintigraphy using a large-field-of-view gamma camera and general-purpose collimator, which was interfaced to a computer, was performed for the initial 20 min without a diuretic agent. The data collection protocol was 1-s interval images for the initial 1 min followed by 10-s interval images for 19 min in 64×64 matrix. Background corrected time-activity curves were generated from regions of interest placed over both the kidneys with background around them. The renal split function (RSF) and glomerular filtration rate (GFR) were calculated from a regression equation obtained between creatinine clearance and the initial 2- to 3-min uptake of ^{99m}Tc-DTPA [5]. The patient was instructed to void and thereafter furosemide at a dose of 0.4 mg/kg (with a maximal dose of 20 mg) was given intravenously 2 min after the initiation of the diuretic data collection. The data were collected at 10-s interval images for 15 min. The

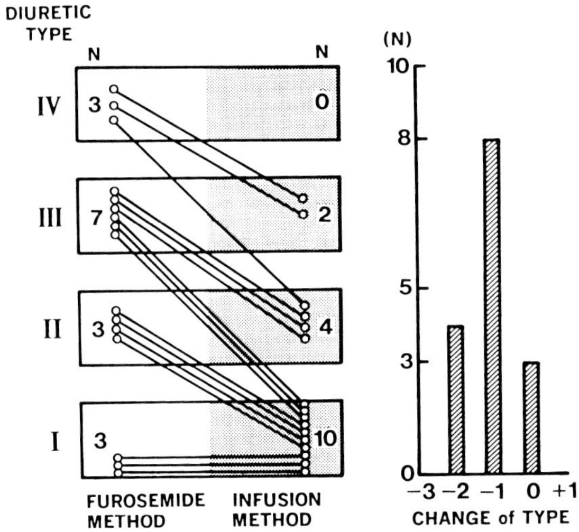

Fig. 1. Comparison of diuresis between furosemide diuretic renography and direct infusion renography. In the infusion study, none of the patients showed a completely obstructed type of diuresis curve.

background corrected time-activity curves of the diuresis washout phase also were generated and a clearance half-time ($D\text{-}T_{1/2}$) was calculated from monoexponential curve fitting by the least square method [8]. The patency of the upper urinary system was categorized with $D\text{-}T_{1/2}$. Type I (normal) was shorter than 10 min in $D\text{-}T_{1/2}$. Type II (equivocal) was between 10 and 20 min in $D\text{-}T_{1/2}$. Type III (partially obstructed) was longer than 20 min in $D\text{-}T_{1/2}$. Type IV (completely obstructed) increased with time.

The patients visited for further evaluation of urinary drainage by direct infusion renography within 7 days after the conventional diuretic renography. ^{99m}Tc-DTPA at a dose of 18.5–37 MBq was injected through the catheter and thereafter normal saline was infused at 3 drops/s. The data were recorded at the beginning of the infusion at 1-s interval frames for 15 min. $D\text{-}T_{1/2}$ was calculated in the same way as in the furosemide diuresis.

Results

In conventional furosemide renography, there were 3 patients who showed a completely obstructed curve. They were converted to type III in 2 kidneys and type II in 1 by the infusion technique. The remaining 12 patients also fell into lower types of diuresis curves on the infusion study (fig. 1). There were no patients who showed more prolonged clearance half-time on the conventional diuretic renography than on the direct infusion renography. The regression equation between $D\text{-}T_{1/2}$ of furosemide renography (X) and of infusion renography (Y) was $Y = 1.44 \pm 0.17X$

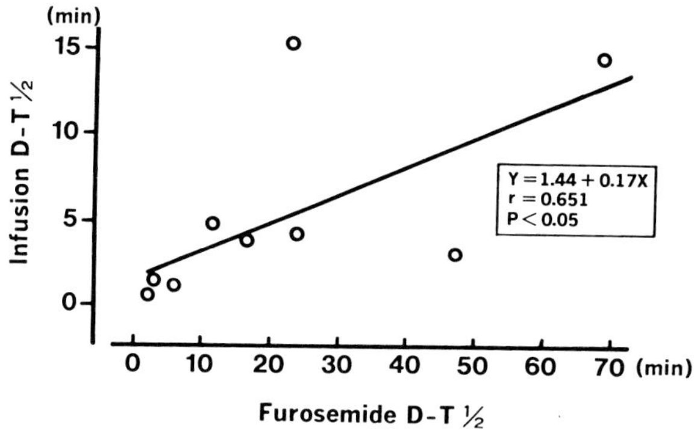

Fig. 2. Scattered diagram of a clearance half-time (D-$T_{1/2}$) between furosemide diuretic renography and direct infusion renography in the patients without complete obstruction on furosemide diuresis renography.

($r = 0.651$, $p < 0.05$) (fig. 2). We compared between renal split glomerular function and clearance half-time on furosemide-augmented renography in 8 kidneys and found no significant correlation between them.

A Case Report

A 7-year-old boy was admitted with left hydronephrosis (fig. 3). The standard renal scintigraphy showed decreased renal parenchymal uptake of ^{99m}Tc-DTPA and thin cortical image suggestive of marked dilatation of the pelvicalyceal systems on the left kidney. Calculated GFR of both kidneys was 71 ml/min and the left RSF was 30.4%. Furosemide renography showed no urinary drainage through the upper urinary systems, categorized as type IV. Infusion renography performed 3 days later showed the presence of the upper urinary patency, categorized as type II. Pyeloplasty was carried out due to the congenital pelviureteric junction stenosis.

Discussion

It has been agreed generally that furosemide-augmented diuresis renography is the initial procedure to distinguish between a dilated and obstructed urinary tract that requires an operation, and a dilated but nonobstructed urinary system that requires no surgical manipulation [4, 7, 9, 10]. However, several clinical factors have been observed to give false-positive and false-negative results [2, 6, 8, 10]. In a physiologic aspect, diuresis may be separated to two responding processes: the first response is related to the function of the kidney and the second response is related to the physical and mechanical ability of the urinary tract transporting the urine into the urinary bladder. The renal split function, the state of

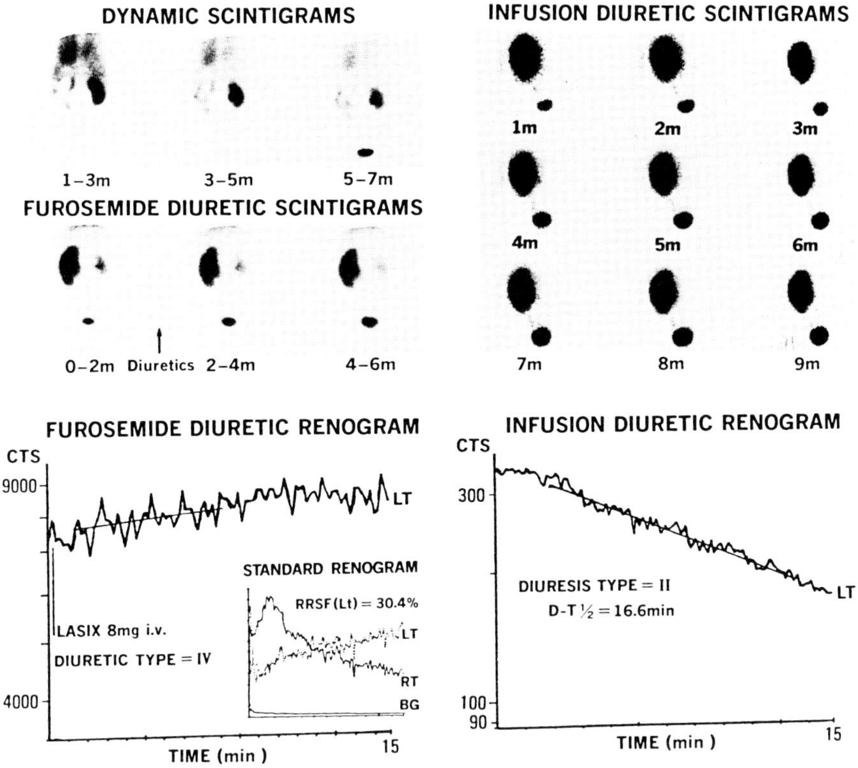

Fig. 3. Furosemide-augmented renography and infusion renography in a 7-year-old boy with hydronephrosis of the left kidney (see text).

hydration, and the dose of diuretic injected are the factors which influence the urinary output from the renal parenchyma to the upper urinary collecting systems. The other factors such as the volume capacity of the urinary tract, ureteric stricture, loss of physical contraction of the smooth muscle and the intravesical pressure may contribute the urine transport through the urinary tract.

Because infusion renography can overshadow the influence of diuresis to the functional responses of the renal parenchyma, we compared two different diuresis renographies: the conventional furosemide method and the direct intrapelvic infusion method. The purpose of the study was not to compare which of the techniques was more suitable for evaluating urinary patency, but to clarify whether conventional furosemide intervention could induce sufficient diuresis to drain the urine collected in the dilated urinary tract. The results in the present study indicate that conventional diuretic renography cannot provide sufficient urinary washout to transfer the urine collected in the dilated urinary systems. In order to diminish the incidence of false-positive responses by furosemide renography, enforced diuresis must be attempted to maintain intrapelvic compliance sufficient enough to transfer urinary washout from the urinary tract. From the regression equation obtained in this study, we presume that diuresis by the conventional method is grossly about 3–6 times less effective than that by the infusion method. Volume expansion diuretic renography [1] seems to be a good attempt to accelerate diuresis. Direct intrapelvic infusion diuresis renography may be helpful to estimate the superiority of a newly applied diuresis method.

References

1 Howman-Giles R, Uren R, Roy LR, et al: Volume expansion diuretic renal scan in urinary tract obstruction. J Nucl Med 1987;28:824–828.
2 Hunter GJ, Gordon J, Sweeney L, et al: ^{99m}Tc-DTPA scanning with diuretic washout. Is it useful in the investigation of obstruction in the presence of gross renal tract dilatation? Br J Urol 1987;59:208–210.
3 Ireton RC, Parker RM: Diuretic renography in evaluating dilated upper urinary tract in children. Urology 1987;29:178–184.
4 Itoh K, Imanaka K, Nonomura K, et al: Clinical evaluation of diuretic renography in obstructive uropathy. Kaku-igaku 1982;19:721–732.
5 Itoh K, Arakawa M: Re-estimation of renal function with ^{99m}Tc-DTPA by the Gates method. Kaku-igaku 1987;24:389–396.
6 Kass EJ, Majd M, Belma AB: Comparison of the diuretic renography and the pressure perfusion study in children. J Urol 1985;134:92–95.
7 Koff SA, Thrall JH, Keyes JW Jr: Diuretic radionuclide urography. A non-invasive method for evaluating nephroureteral dilatation. J Urol 1979;122:451–454.
8 Krueger RP, Ash JM, Silver MM, et al: Primary hydronephrosis. Assesment of diuretic renography, pelvis perfusion pressure, operative findings, and renal and ureteral history. Urol Clin N Am 1980;7:231–242.
9 O'Reilly PH, Testa HJ, Lawson DJ, et al: Diuresis renography in equivocal tract obstruction. Br J Urol 1978;50:76–80.
10 O'Reilly PH: Diuresis renography 8 years later. An update. J Urol 1986;136:993–999.

Dr. Kazuo Itoh, Department of Nuclear Medicine, Hokkaido University School of Medicine, Kita-15, Nishi-7, Kita-ku, Sapporo 060 (Japan)

Blaufox MD, Hollenberg NK, Raynaud C (eds): Radionuclides in Nephro-Urology.
Contrib Nephrol. Basel, Karger, 1990, vol 79, pp 161–165

Serial Furosemide Renography in Asymptomatic Hydronephrosis Diagnosed by Ultrasound in utero and Neonatally

H.S. Clarke, M.M. DeBeukelaer, K.A. Kropp, R.R. Lenke, W.H. Persutte, W.J. Potvin

Medical College of Ohio, Toledo, Ohio, USA

Hydronephrosis secondary to ureteropelvic junction obstruction, the most common form of urinary tract obstruction in children, has recently undergone significant change in its clinical presentation. Ten to 15 years ago what was most often discovered during the routine work-up for a urinary tract infection or as a palpable abdominal mass in an older child, is now often identified in utero during maternal ultrasonography. The number of infants that exhibit some degree of hydronephrosis during gestation has been reported as high as 1 in 1,000 [1].

The early detection of asymptomatic hydronephrosis has stimulated renewed interest in the pathophysiologic mechanisms causing this entity as well as debate over its management. Some investigators advocate surgical correction at the earliest opportunity for maximum preservation of renal function [2–4]. Others take the position that early intervention is of no increased benefit, and many of these infants have a mild, or transient obstruction that may resolve, and therefore only require careful observation [5–7]. This paper summarizes our experience over the past 5 years with 16 infants referred for evaluation of asymptomatic hydronephrosis.

Materials and Methods

From 1983 to 1989, 32 infants were referred to the Division of Pediatric Nephrology at the Medical College of Ohio Hospital for evaluation of hydronephrosis, diagnosed on maternal ultrasound in 24 and neonatally in 8 (< 4 weeks of age). All infants underwent repeat ultrasound and voiding cystourethrogram or nuclear cystography to rule out vesicoureteral reflux. Some underwent excretory urogram (IVP) or CT scan to rule out other anomalies. Sixteen infants were found to have other anomalies or significant vesicoureteral reflux and were excluded. The remaining 16 infants were found to have asymptomatic hydronephrosis. These 16 infants underwent a ^{99m}Tc-DTPA renal perfusion study followed by a ^{131}I-hippuran renogram. Those infants that demonstrated an obstructive pattern on the renogram had their renogram repeated with furosemide stimulation (1 mg/kg i.v.). Patients were referred at varying times during this protocol for surgical intervention. Most recently over the past 2 years patients with a persistent obstructive pattern on furosemide renography at 6 months of age have been referred for surgical repair.

The current protocol for the nuclear medicine studies is as follows: The patient is brought to the hospital short-stay unit. An IV is established and the patient is hydrated, sedated with chloral hydrate and a Foley catheter is placed. The infant is then transported to the nuclear medicine department and a ^{99m}Tc-DTPA perfusion study followed by a ^{131}I-hippuran renogram is performed. This initial renogram curve is analyzed and if there is an obstructive pattern, as defined by a $T_{1/2}$ maximum activity of greater than 8 min, a repeat renogram is performed with the injection of furosemide (1 mg/kg i.v.) at the time where maximum activity was achieved on the prior study. Infants that demonstrate normal excretory function with furosemide stimulation are followed with repeat studies at 1, 3 and 6 months of age and then on a yearly basis. Infants that demonstrate a pattern of obstruction have repeat studies performed in a similar fashion with additional studies as indicated on an individual case basis.

Results

Of the 16 infants with asymptomatic hydronephrosis, 12 were male, 11 had unilateral hydronephrosis and 5 had bilateral hydronephrosis. Two patients with bilateral hydronephrosis diagnosed in utero were found to have unilateral hydronephrosis on postnatal ultrasound exam. The infants were classified in two groups based on the results of the initial furosemide renogram.

Those that showed a return to one half maximum activity within 8 min or less were classified as nonobstructed (group I, n = 11) (fig. 1a, b). Those infants that had an initial furosemide renogram with a return to one half maximum activity in greater than 8 min were classified as obstructed (group II, n = 5) (fig. 2a). All patients had abnormal renograms initially. Of the group I infants, 4 improved on subsequent renograms to the extent that they no longer required furosemide renography. Ultrasound in this group demonstrated persistent hydronephrosis in 9 and improvement in 2. All patients in group II demonstrated a furosemide renogram that remained elevated on one or more sequential studies. All were referred for surgical evaluation based on these findings. One patient early in the study underwent unilateral dismembered pyeloplasty at 2 months of age for ureteropelvic junction obstruction. Two others had similar ureteropelvic junction obstruction repaired at 6 months of age and of the remaining 2 patients, 1 is scheduled for surgical repair and the other has improved on a 6-month furosemide renogram and has had surgery deferred (fig. 2b). Three patients have had postoperative follow-up

a

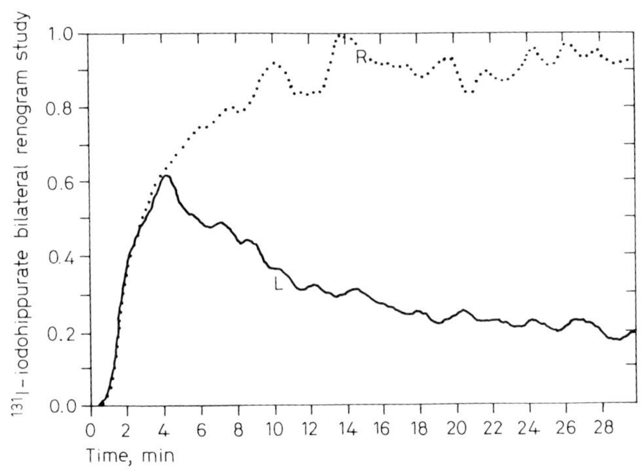

b

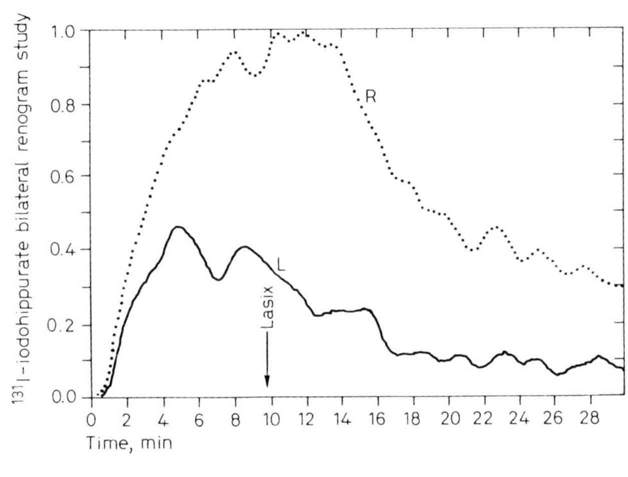

Fig. 1. a ^{131}I-hippuran renogram in a group I infant showing an obstructive pattern in the right kidney. *b* ^{131}I-hippuran renogram in the same infant with furosemide stimulation showing a good response.

renograms with and without furosemide as well as follow-up ultrasound. The postoperative renograms remain abnormal while the furosemide renograms normalized in all 3 of these patients. Pre- and postoperative ultrasound showed persistent hydronephrosis. Neither group showed significant differences in renal function, growth pattern, blood pressure or complication rate.

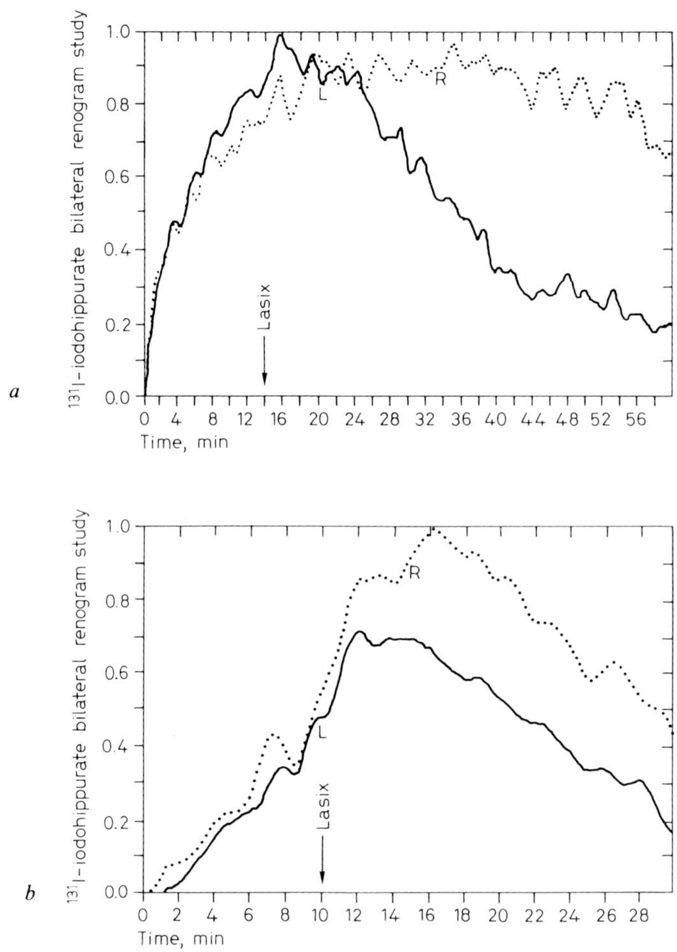

Fig. 2. a Initial furosemide-stimulated ^{131}I-hippuran renogram in a group II infant showing no response in the right kidney. *b* Furosemide-stimulated renogram in same infant at 6 months, showing an improved response.

Discussion

With the advent of sophisticated prenatal ultrasound screening there has been a large increase in the number of genitourinary anomalies being detected in utero. As a consequence of this, many more infants are being referred for evaluation of hydronephrosis than in previous years. The management of this clinical entity has undergone considerable evolution over the past several years and our experience mirrors this change in management. Many centers initially advocated intervention at the earliest possible time to preserve renal functional mass. Indeed, King et al. [2] and others [3] support this position with their data which shows that there is no increase in morbidity or mortality in neonatal dismembered pyeloplasty for repair of ureteropelvic junction obstruction compared to older children. More recently there is increasing support for close observation in conjunction with serial diuretic renography. This is our current view as well as others [5–8] and is based on the concept that many of these infants have a transient form of hydronephrosis that remains stable in most cases and spontaneously improves in others. This is illustrated in the two group II infants in our study who have not as yet undergone surgery. One has improved and the second, while not showing improvement, has not shown any deterioration in renal function.

In conclusion, diuresis renography can readily separate those infants, without obstruction, that can be conservatively managed (group I). Serial furosemide renograms may also aid in detecting mild or improving hydronephrosis that does not require surgical intervention. And finally, serial furosemide renograms showing no improvement may indicate the need for surgical repair prior to the occurrence of any deterioration in renal function.

References

1 Helin I, Persson PH: Prenatal diagnosis of urinary tract abnormalities by ultrasound. Pediatrics 1986;78:879.
2 King LR, Coughlin PW, Bloch EC, et al: The case for immediate pyeloplasty in the neonate with ureteropelvic junction obstruction. J Urol 1984;132:725.
3 Mandel J: Early postnatal reconstruction of UPJ obstruction diagnosed in utero. Dial Pediatr Urol 1986;8:3.
4 Bejjani B, Belman B: Ureteropelvic junction obstruction in newborns and infants. J Urol 1982;128:770.
5 Koff SA, Hayden LJ, Cirulli C, et al: Pathophysiology of ureteropelvic junction obstruction: Experimental and clinical observations. J Urol 1986;136:336.
6 Bernstein GT, Mandell J, Lebowitz RL et al: Ureteropelvic junction obstruction in the neonate. J Urol 1988;140:216.
7 Homsy YL, Williot P, Danais S: Transitional neonatal hydronephrosis: Fact or fancy? J Urol 1986;136:339.
8 Piepsz A, Hall M, Ham HR, et al: Prospective management of neonates with pelvi-ureteric junction stenosis. Scand J Urol Nephrol 1989;23:31.

M. M. De Beukelaer MD, Department of Pediatrics, Medical College of Ohio,
PO Box 10008, Toledo, OH 43699 (USA)

Blaufox MD, Hollenberg NK, Raynaud C (eds): Radionuclides in Nephro-Urology.
Contrib Nephrol. Basel, Karger, 1990, vol 79, pp 166–169

DMSA Studies in Infants under One Year of Age

Monica A. Rossleigh, Meredith J. Wilson, Andrew R. Rosenberg, Barry S. Elison, Sue Cahill, Robert H. Farnsworth

Department of Nuclear Medicine, Prince of Wales Hospital, and Departments of Nephrology and Urology, Prince of Wales Children's Hospital, Sydney, N.S.W., Australia

Renal scarring is an important sequela of urinary tract infection (UTI) because of the risk of subsequent renal impairment and the possible development of systemic hypertension. Technetium-99m dimercaptosuccinic acid (DMSA) is an excellent cortical scanning agent, which localizes in the proximal tubular cells with only minimal excretion and thus allows visualization of functioning renal parenchyma [1]. It is considered the scanning agent of choice to demonstrate postinflammatory renal scars [2]. In this paper, we report the results of DMSA studies performed in infants under 1 year of age at risk of renal scarring.

Materials and Methods

DMSA renal studies were performed in 63 infants under 1 year of age undergoing urological assessment – 49 had presented with UTI; in 14 the assessment was carried out for other reasons. All patients underwent intravenous urography (IVU) and micturating cystograms. The clinical history was noted in each case.

The DMSA studies were performed 3 h following the intravenous injection of 40 MBq ^{99m}Tc-DMSA on a GE 400 AT gamma camera connected to an MDS A_2 computer. Standard posterior planar views were collected for 5 min. Posterior pinhole views were also performed for 100,000 counts/kidney. In addition, some patients underwent SPECT examination. This was collected on a 64 × 64 byte matrix during a 360° circular orbit with 64 images collected at 30 s/image. The study was reconstructed in coronal, sagittal and transaxial planes with slices of 1 pixel width. Differential renal function was calculated from the posterior planar data.

The diagnostic criteria used for reporting renal cortical abnormalities on the DMSA studies were: reduction in kidney function and/or decreased or absent uptake of tracer in the renal cortex causing distortion or indentation of the normal renal outline [3].

The time interval between the UTI and the subsequent DMSA study was greater than 3 months in 30 of 49 patients and greater than 1 month in 47 of 49 patients, thus reducing the potentially reversible effect of acute infection on the DMSA study [4]. The time interval

Table 1. Results of IVP and DMSA studies

	Normal IVP		Abnormal IVP	
	UTI	reflux no UTI	UTI	reflux no UTI
Normal DMSA	23	10	0	0
Abnormal DMSA	18	4	8	0

between the IVU and DMSA study was less than 3 months in 50 of the 63 patients and less than 6 months in 59 of the 63 patients. The IVU was performed before the DMSA in all but 2 patients.

Results

The results are summarized in table 1. In the 49 patients with a history of UTI, 26 had renal cortical abnormalities detected on the DMSA study and 8 had changes of reflux nephropathy on IVU. All infants with abnormal IVU findings had corresponding abnormalities on the DMSA study. Seven of the 8 patients with abnormal IVU had a greater than 22% difference in differential function, as assessed by DMSA (range 22–80%). Of the other 14 infants with reflux but no history of UTI, 4 had abnormal DMSA scans and none had IVU changes of reflux nephropathy.

Abnormal DMSA scans were seen more frequently in association with higher grades of reflux. In the UTI group, there was no apparent difference in the incidence of DMSA abnormality between those infants presenting with fever (21/58 kidneys abnormal) and those without fever (12/40 kidneys abnormal). Our results, however, suggest an association between the occurrence of UTI in the neonatal period and increased rate of scarring, infants presenting under 1 month of age having a 50% incidence of scarred kidneys compared to infants presenting over 6 months of age having a 17% incidence of scarred kidneys.

Discussion

Our data indicates that DMSA renal studies appear to be more sensitive than IVU in the early detection of renal scarring in infants (fig. 1). As all infants, but 1, with abnormal IVU had a greater than 22% difference in differential function as assessed by DMSA, this suggests that a signifi-

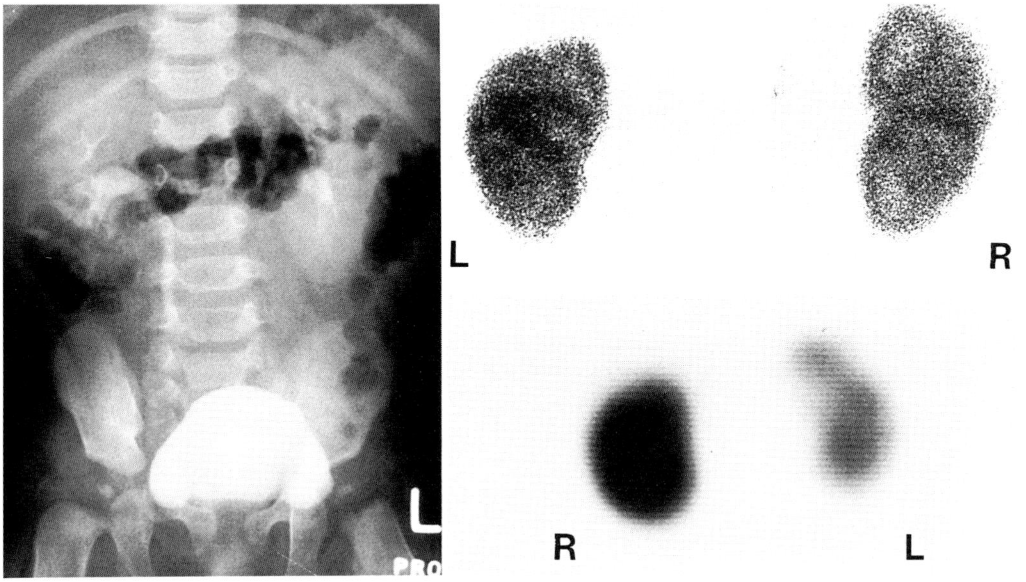

a b c

Fig. 1. a Normal IVP in an infant presenting with UTI and fever. Micturating cystogram showed bilateral grade III reflux. *b* Pinhole views of the DMSA study performed on the same infant demonstrate absent uptake in a wedge-shaped pattern in the left upper pole. *c* The SPECT study confirmed an area of cortical loss in the left upper pole laterally, shown here on a coronal slice.

cant amount of renal cortical damage must be present before a scar can be detected on IVU.

There was no relationship between the presence of fever in an infant with UTI and the risk of renal scarring. In addition, our results suggest an association between early occurrence of UTI and the risk of scarring.

There was an increasing incidence of DMSA abnormality with increasing grade of reflux. In addition, the presence of abnormal DMSA studies in some infants without UTI suggests that renal scarring may occur with sterile vesicoureteric reflux.

References

1 Bingham JB, Maisey MN: An evaluation of the use of ^{99m}Tc-dimercaptosuccinic acid (DMSA) as a static renal imaging agent. Br J Radiol 1978;51:559–607.

2 Merrick BM, Uttley WS, Wild SR: The detection of pyelonephritic scarring in children by radioisotope imaging. Br J Radiol 1980;53:544–556.

3 Wujanto R, Testa HJ, Shields RA, et al: Assessment of Renal Function and Scarring: Is a DMSA Scan Always Necessary? Contr Nephrol. Basel, Karger, 1987, vol 56, pp 250–255.
4 Rushton HG, Majd M, Chandra R, et al: Evaluation of ^{99m}technetium-dimercapto-succinic acid renal scans in experimental acute pyelonephritis in piglets. J Urol 1988;140:1169–1174.

Dr. Monica A. Rossleigh, Nuclear Medicine Department,
Prince of Wales Hospital, Randwick, NSW 2031 (Australia)

Blaufox MD, Hollenberg NK, Raynaud C (eds): Radionuclides in Nephro-Urology.
Contrib Nephrol. Basel, Karger, 1990, vol 79, pp 170–175

Paradoxical Increased Glucoheptonate Uptake in Experimental Renovascular Hypertension

H.B. Lee, B. Gale, M.D. Blaufox
Albert Einstein College of Medicine, Bronx, N.Y., USA

Angiotensin-converting enzyme (ACE) inhibitors have the potential to disturb the balance between the pressure and blood flow required to maintain glomerular filtration rate in renal artery stenosis (RAS). ACE inhibition results in a reduction of glomerular filtration rate and renal blood flow in the kidney with RAS. These physiological effects after ACE inhibition potentially provide greater sensitivity for the diagnosis of RAS than conventional renography. However, ACE inhibitors may affect glomerular filtration rate and renal blood flow differently depending on the dose administered and the degree of the RAS [1–3]. Experiments both in patients and animals suggest that glomerular filtration after ACE inhibition decreases in the kidney with RAS while glomerular filtration rate in the normal kidney usually is not changed [2–4].

^{99m}Tc-DTPA is useful to measure glomerular filtration rate and ^{131}I-OIH provides an accurate estimate of effective renal plasma flow (ERPF). Radiotracer uptake with these agents shows asymmetry between kidneys with RAS and those with normal renal arteries. ^{99m}Tc-glucoheptonate (^{99m}Tc-GHA) is a radiopharmaceutical agent partly filtered by the glomerulus and partly retained in the tubule. Its potential role in the differential diagnosis of renovascular hypertension has not been evaluated fully.

Methods

Forty-two Sprague-Dawley male rats weighing 300–320 g were studied 1–2 weeks after the left renal artery was clamped. RAS was produced by clamping the left renal artery with polyethylene tubing (PE 50). Two millimeter lengths of tubing were cut longitudinally and placed over the main renal artery, taking care not to interfere with its branches. The tubing was tied in place with 4-0 or 6-0 surgical silk thread. The rats were maintained on a normal diet with laboratory rat purina chow and provided with water ad libitum. At the time of the study, catheters were placed in the animals' left and right ureter (PE 10 silastic tubing),

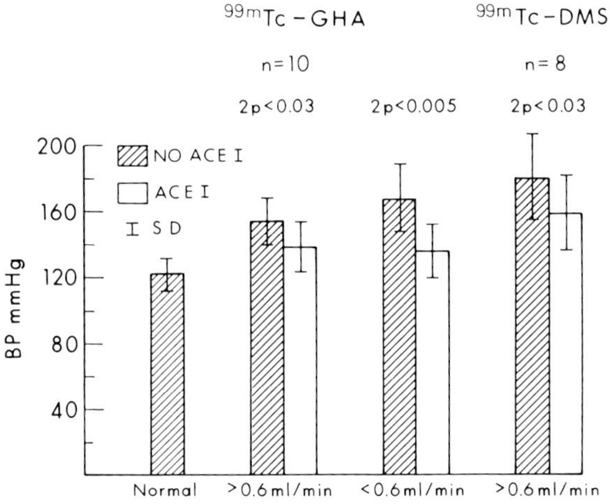

Fig. 1. The mean BP of animals with two normal kidneys and two kidneys one clamped before and after the administration of ACE inhibition is shown on the bar graph. The BPs in the animals with RAS are all significantly higher than in the control animals. Although the degree of change varied, it was significantly decreased in each group.

femoral vein and femoral artery (PE 50). Blood pressure (BP) was recorded on a Hewlett-Packard 78205 D recorder using a femoral artery catheter. ^{131}I-OIH in saline (20 μCi/ml) was infused at 1.5 ml/h using the femoral vein catheters. ERPF was determined every 5 min for 2–3 times using a continuous infusion method. Captopril (1.3–1.7 mg/100 g b.w.) was administered after the control ERPF measurement. After the BP was stabilized at the new level, ERPF was determined again as described above. Immediately after ERPF determination, 50 μCi of ^{99m}Tc-GHA in 0.1 ml was injected via the femoral vein. Three minutes after the ^{99m}Tc-GHA administration, sodium pentobarbital (0.13 mg) was injected via the femoral artery. The kidneys were removed immediately and weighed.

The rats were divided into two groups for analysis based on the function of the clamped kidney (ClK) before the ACE inhibition: mild renal function reduction and severe renal function reduction. The group of animals whose initial ERPF of the ClK was > 0.6 ml/min/100 g b.w. was considered to have mild renal function reduction and those whose initial ERPF of ClK was < 0.6 ml/min/100 g b.w. were considered to have severe renal function reduction. ^{99m}Tc-GHA uptake data were compared between these groups of animals, including those that did not receive captopril and those that did receive captopril. Data were analyzed with a group t test using 2p values for levels of significance.

Results

Rats with two normal kidneys had significantly lower mean BP (123 ± 9 (SD) mm Hg, n = 10) than rats with two kidneys one clamped (169 ± 2, $2p < 0.0005$, n = 42). BP decreased significantly in all groups after ACE inhibition (fig. 1). In the ^{99m}Tc-GHA study group, the animals with

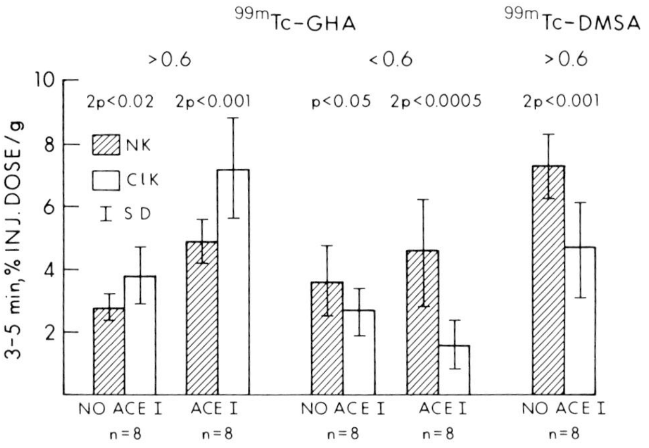

Fig. 2. Total kidney uptake of ^{99m}Tc-GHA and ^{99m}Tc-DMSA are compared before and after ACE inhibition. ^{99m}Tc-GHA uptake in the ClK was significantly higher than normal kidney, but ^{99m}Tc-DMSA in the ClK was lower than normal kidney.

mild RAS decreased BP after ACE inhibition from 155 ± 15 to 136 ± 15 (SD) mm Hg ($2p < 0.005$). In the ^{99m}Tc-DMSA study group, the animals with mild RAS decreased BP after ACE inhibition from 171 ± 26 to 139 ± 23 mm Hg ($2p < 0.03$).

^{99m}Tc-GHA uptake in the ClK (mild reduction) was 3.77 ± 0.33% (SE) injected dose per gram of tissue with no ACE inhibition. ^{99m}Tc-GHA uptake was significantly lower in the NK (2.77 ± 0.14, $2p < 0.02$) than the ClK in this group. In the ACE-inhibited group, ^{99m}Tc-GHA uptake in the ClK (7.17 ± 0.51) was significantly higher than NK (4.89 ± 0.24, $2p < 0.005$). Unlike the ^{99m}Tc-GHA study, ^{99m}Tc-DMSA uptake [unpubl. data] in the ClK (4.75 ± 0.64) was significantly lower than in the NK (7.27 ± 0.40, $2p < 0.005$) (fig. 2). In the baseline study without ACE inhibitors in the severely reduced function group ^{99m}Tc-GHA uptake in the ClK (2.66 ± 0.31) was lower than the NK (3.75 ± 0.46, NS). In the ACE-inhibited group, ^{99m}Tc uptake in the ClK (1.60 ± 0.28) was significantly lower than in the NK (4.55 ± 0.59, $2p < 0.0005$).

Pre-captopril ERPF in the mildly impaired group was 1.01 ± 0.19 in ClK and 1.38 ± 0.35 in NK ($2p < 0.002$), and post-captopril was 0.58 ± 0.4 in ClK and 1.18 ± 0.42 in NK ($2p < 0.005$). Pre- and post-ERPF in the ClK was significantly different ($2p < 0.007$) but ERPF did not change significantly in the NK (fig. 3). Pre- and post-captopril ERPF in the animals with severely impaired renal function in the ClK was 0.39 ± 0.06 and 0.10 ± 0.03 ($2p < 0.001$) respectively, and ERPF in the NK was

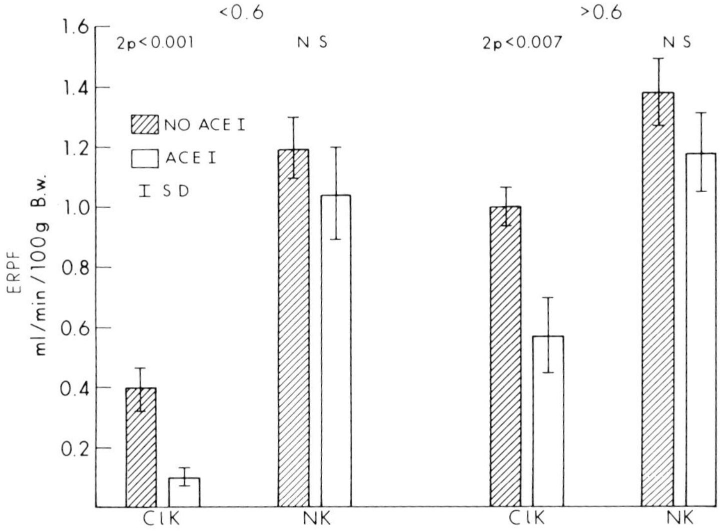

Fig. 3. ^{131}I-OIH clearance of ClK and normal kidney are compared before and after ACE inhibition. The ClK ^{131}I-OIH clearance was decreased significantly by the ACE inhibition but normal kidney clearance did not change.

1.19 ± 0.12 and 1.04 ± 0.16 (NS). ERPF in the ClK was significantly lower than in the NK both pre-captopril ($2p < 0.005$) and post-captopril ($2p < 0.005$).

Discussion

Nuclear medicine techniques are useful for the measurement of split renal function. A significant fraction of the injected dose of ^{99m}Tc-radiotracer is retained in the cortex but reported values vary [5–9]. Although ^{99m}Tc-GHA accumulates continuously for some period of time in the kidney, its 1–3 min and 2–4 h accumulation correlate well in patients and in animal studies [5] when the data from the kidney with RAS are not included.

In the present study, 3–5 min ^{99m}Tc-GHA uptake values were measured. Ten out of 16 rats in the control group had a higher ^{99m}Tc-GHA uptake in the ClK than the NK when the animals were not analyzed on the basis of mild or severe reduction in renal function of the ClK. Nine out of 18 rats in the captopril-inhibited group had a higher ^{99m}Tc-GHA uptake in the ClK than NK. These results are more clear after the animals were differentiated by the initial ERPF of ClK. All 8 animals had higher ^{99m}Tc-GHA uptake in the ClK than the NK in the ERPF > 0.6 group and 2 out of 8 animals had higher ^{99m}Tc-GHA uptake in the ClK than the NK in the group with severe RAS. Among the captopril-treated group, 9 out of 10 animals had higher ^{99m}Tc-GHA uptake in the ClK than the NK in the animals with mild RAS and all 8 animals had lower ^{99m}Tc-GHA uptake in the ClK than the NK among the severe stenosis group. The relative difference of ^{99m}Tc-GHA uptake between the ClK and the NK was greater in the captopril-treated group ($2p < 0.005$) than control group ($2p < 0.02$) in those animals with mild RAS and the animals with severe RAS changed more significantly after ACE inhibition ($2p < 0.0005$).

Creatinine and inulin clearances in 2 dogs were compared using quantitative differential functions tests of ^{99m}Tc-GHA by other investigators in another study. The percent difference between the ClK and the NK was estimated. When the ^{99m}Tc-GHA method was used, the ClK renal function was higher than the NK. Considering that the creatinine clearance in ClK in these 2 animals was 39.3 and 45.1% of the total clearances, the renal function in these kidneys was mildly reduced by the RAS. The author attributed the higher results of ^{99m}Tc-GHA to the shielding effect of the liver [10].

The paradoxically increased ^{99m}Tc-GHA observed in this study is difficult to explain. It is unlikely in this very short time period that it is due to retention of urine. Although a mechanism for this observation has not been identified, it is important to note the potential error of evaluating patients with RAS using ^{99m}Tc-GHA. A falsely elevated uptake on the affected side might make an accurate diagnosis difficult. This possibility should be evaluated in humans before using ^{99m}Tc-GHA for the differential diagnosis of patients with RVH.

References

1 Lee HB, Blaufox MD: Differential effect of captopril on GFR in rats with renovascular hypertension. J Nucl Med 1985;26:72.

2 Oei HY, Geyskes GG, Mees Dorhout EJ, et al: The significance of captopril renography in renovascular hypertension; in Blaufox MD (ed): Contr Nephrol Basel, Karger, 1987, vol 56, pp 95–103.

3 Sfakianakis GN, Bourgoignie JJ, Jaffe D, et al: Single-dose captopril scintigraphy in the diagnosis of renovascular hypertension. J Nucl Med 1987;28:1383–1392.

4 Lee HB, Blaufox MD: Renal functional changes after converting enzyme inhibition or nitroprusside in hypertensive rats; in Blaufox MD (ed): Contr Nephrol Basel, Karger, 1987 vol 56, pp 87–94.

5 Ziessman HA, Balseiro J, Fahey FH, et al: ^{99m}Tc-glucoheptonate for quantitation of differential renal function. Am J Roentgenol 1978;148:665–668.

6 Enlander D, Weber PM, dos Remedios LV: Renal cortical imaging in 35 patients. Superior quality with ^{99m}Tc-DMSA. J Nucl Med 1974;15:743–749.
7 Lee HB, Blaufox MD: Mechanism of renal concentrations of technetium 99m-glucoheptonate. J Nucl Med 1985;26:1308–1313.
8 Yee CA, Lee HB, Blaufox MD: ^{99m}Tc-DMSA renal uptake. Influence of biochemical and physiologic factors. J Nucl Med 1982;22:1054–1058.
9 Arnold RW, Subramanian G, McAfee JG, et al: Comparison of ^{99m}Tc-complex. J Nucl Med 1975;16:359–369.
10 Corriere JN, Staum MM, Godbois WF: Technetium-99m stannous glucoheptonate for renal imaging and evaluating individual renal function. Surg Forum 1975;26:582–584.

H.B. Lee, MD, Department of Nuclear Medicine, Montefiore Medical Center,
Albert Einstein College of Medicine, 1300 Morris Park Avenue,
Bronx, NY 10461 (USA)

Blaufox MD, Hollenberg NK, Raynaud C (eds): Radionuclides in Nephro-Urology.
Contrib Nephrol. Basel, Karger, 1990, vol 79, pp 176–180

Captopril-Stimulated Renography versus Renal Vein Renins in Two-Kidney, Two-Clip Hypertension

Joseph V. Nally, Jr., Luis A. Bedoya, Chan H. Park, Arturo Martinez, Nicholas T. Stowe[1]

The Cleveland Clinic Foundation, Cleveland, Ohio, USA

Renovascular hypertension (RVHT) remains the subject of active investigation with the hopes of identifying patients with potentially correctable hypertension and preserving their renal function. Captopril renography continues to enjoy its ascendancy as a diagnostic modality in this area. However, the majority of diagnostic studies have focused upon unilateral renal artery stenosis (RAS) – the classical model of renin-dependent hypertension. Debate exists over the renin dependency of individual kidney function and the concomitant hypertension in bilateral RAS. Traditionally, the clinician has relied upon invasive renal vein renin (RVR) determinations to address these issues.

The purpose of this study was to examine the effect of angiotensin-converting enzyme (ACE) inhibition with captopril upon renal function, RVRs and renography, using ^{99m}Tc-diethylenetriaminepentaacetic acid (Tc-DTPA) and ^{131}I-orthoiodohippurate (hippuran), in a canine model of two-kidney, two-clip (2K, 2C) hypertension. More specifically, our goal was to address two questions: (1) Is captopril renography diagnostic and predictive of the more stenotic kidney in bilateral renal artery disease? (2) Is there a correlation between the noninvasive captopril renography studies and more invasive renal function studies or RVRs?

Methods

Studies were performed in female mongrel dogs (n = 13) who were allowed free access to food and water during the course of the study. For the baseline studies, dogs were anesthetized with pentobarbital (30 mg/kg) and mean arterial pressure (MAP), clearance of inulin

[1] The authors acknowledge the technical expertise of Kathy Butters, CNMT, and the editorial assistance of Ray Borazanian.

Table 1. Renal function and RVR data following RAS before and after captopril

	RAS		RAS + captopril	
	more stenotic kidney	less stenotic kidney	more stenotic kidney	less stenotic kidney
GFR, ml/min	14.6 ± 3.6^{a}	29.1 ± 3.7^{a}	$6.7 \pm 2.0^{a,b}$	$20.7 \pm 4.6^{a,b}$
ERPF, ml/min	64.2 ± 15.2^{a}	135.1 ± 22.1^{a}	$34.7 \pm 12.4^{a,b}$	118.1 ± 22.9^{a}
RVR, ng/ml/h	28.7 ± 9.7	19.1 ± 7.0	$95.2 \pm 22.5^{a,b}$	$46.2 \pm 11.3^{a,b}$

[a] $p < 0.05$ between more and less stenotic kidney.
[b] $p < 0.05$ between pre- and post-captopril in the ipsilateral kidney.

(C_{IN}) and PAH (C_{PAH}) and renography with Tc-DTPA and hippuran were completed, as previously described in our laboratory [1, 2]. The animals were allowed to recover for 5–7 days.

Following recovery, bilateral RAS was created utilizing our metallic vascular clip technique. The stenoses were intentionally asymmetric with a 40–50% stenosis on one side and a 60–80% stenosis of the contralateral artery. On the second postoperative day, renography with Tc-DTPA and hippuran was repeated without captopril. On the following day, the animal was anesthetized for split-function inulin and PAH studies as well as RVR determinations before and after captopril (1.5 mg/kg bolus and 1.5 mg/min infusion). Renography with Tc-DTPA and hippuran was repeated at the conclusion of the clearance studies during captopril infusion.

C_{IN} and C_{PAH} were calculated as an index of glomerular filtration rate (GFR) and effective renal plasma flow (ERPF), respectively. Renin determination was measured by radioimmunoassay. For the renography studies, 5 mCi Tc-DTPA and 50 μCi hippuran dosages were utilized. The studies were performed on a Siemens large field of view gamma camera using a medium-energy collimator with in-house software.

Data is presented as mean ± SEM. Statistical analysis was completed using Student's t test and correlations using SAS.

Results

Poststenosis renal function data (RAS alone) can be seen in table 1. The more severely stenotic kidney (MSSK) was selected as having the lower ERPF prior to captopril infusion. The GFR and ERPF of MSSK were significantly lower (approximately one half) of its contralateral counterpart. The RVRs of MSSK tended to be higher than the less severely stenotic kidney (LSSK) during the pre-captopril periods, but the difference did not achieve statistical significance.

Following captopril administration, there was a significant reduction in MAP (145 ± 5 vs. 116 ± 8 mm Hg, $p < 0.001$). As can be seen in table 1, captopril also resulted in a significant reduction in GFR of both MSSK and LSSK. There was also a significant reduction in ERPF of MSSK, but the

Table 2. ^{99m}Tc-DTPA and ^{131}I-hippuran renographic data before and after captopril

	RAS		RAS + captopril	
	more stenotic kidney	less stenotic kidney	more stenotic kidney	less stenotic kidney
^{99m}-Tc-DTPA				
Uptake, %	43.5 ± 4.5^{b}	56.4 ± 4.5^{b}	$33.1 \pm 5.8^{a,b}$	$66.8 \pm 5.8^{a,b}$
T_{max}, min	2.4 ± 0.4^{b}	1.8 ± 0.2^{b}	7.5 ± 1.8^{b}	6.0 ± 1.7^{b}
	(n = 13)	(n = 13)	(n = 12)	(n = 12)
^{131}I-hippuran				
Uptake, %	37.1 ± 4.0^{a}	62.8 ± 4.0^{a}	29.7 ± 5.1^{a}	70.2 ± 5.1^{a}
T_{max}, min	5.4 ± 1.6^{b}	2.3 ± 0.2^{b}	11.8 ± 1.8^{b}	7.1 ± 1.8^{b}
	(n = 13)	(n = 13)	(n = 11)	(n = 11)

Uptake represents the percent uptake of ^{99m}Tc-DTPA or ^{131}I-hippuran obtained at 40–70 and 0–90 s from the start of the time-activity curves, respectively.
[a] $p < 0.05$ between more and less stenotic kidney.
[b] $p < 0.05$ between pre- and post-captopril in the ipsilateral kidney.

reduction did not reach statistical significance for LSSK. Captopril also induced significant increases in RVRs of each kidney. In addition, the post-captopril RVRs of the MSSK were now significantly higher compared to the LSSK.

The effect of captopril upon the Tc-DTPA and hippuran renograms was assessed visually and quantitatively by analyzing time to maximal activity (T_{max}) and percent relative uptake of each kidney before and after captopril. The effect of captopril could be appreciated equally upon the Tc-DTPA and the hippuran renograms. All renograms changed to some extent after captopril, demonstrating either delayed uptake, delayed excretion, or cortical retention, as defined previously [3]. In 2 of the 13 dogs, the renogram of LSSK did not change with captopril. The effect of captopril upon the quantitative renographic data can be found in table 2. Captopril prolonged the T_{max} of both the MSSK and LSSK in both the Tc-DTPA and hippuran studies. However, captopril resulted in a significant reduction in percent relative uptake in Tc-DTPA of MSSK only.

There were three important correlations of the noninvasive renography studies versus renal function/RVRs following captopril administration. In MSSK only, the reduction in percent uptake with Tc-DTPA correlated with the fall in GFR (fig. 1). Also, only seen with MSSK, the lower percent uptake with both Tc-DTPA and hippuran correlated inversely with post-captopril RVRs (fig. 2a, b).

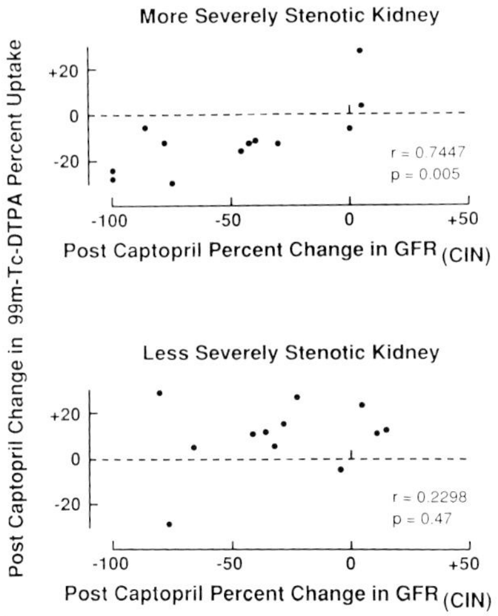

1

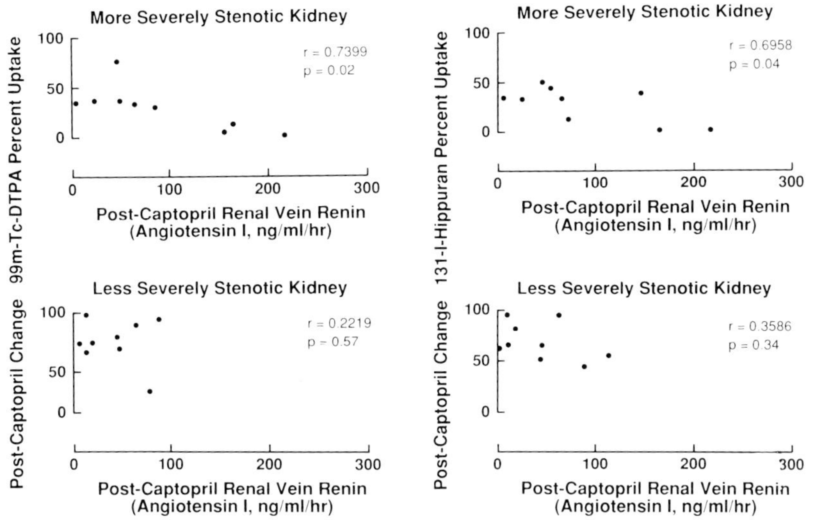

2a 2b

Fig. 1. Correlation between post-captopril change in Tc-DTPA percent uptake and percent change in GFR.

Fig. 2. Correlation between post-captopril Tc-DTPA *(a)* and ^{131}I-hippuran *(b)* percent uptake and post-captopril RVRs.

Discussion

ACE inhibition with captopril resulted in a significant reduction in MAP and GFR of each kidney in our model of 2K, 2C hypertension. In addition, captopril produced a significant rise in RVR determination and altered the renograms of the stenotic kidneys. These changes are consistent with the physiological response observed after captopril administration in human and experimental models of unilateral RAS [1–3]. Earlier studies from our laboratory suggested that such changes were specific for the effects of ACE inhibition upon the stenotic kidney as the renographic alterations were not seen when MAP was lowered with the vasodilator nitroprusside. The current studies demonstrate that angiotensin II plays an important role in maintaining MAP and kidney function in a model of bilateral RAS.

These studies serve to highlight both the effects of captopril upon both the Tc-DTPA and hippuran renograms and the correlations of the captopril-stimulated noninvasive radionuclide studies with more invasive renal function studies and RVR determinations. In the MSSK, ACE inhibition with captopril resulted in a reduction in percent Tc-DTPA uptake which correlated with the percent reduction in GFR and the stimulation of RVR of that kidney. Therefore, the changes in Tc-DTPA uptake, GFR and RVR following captopril administration were lateralized to the MSSK. It is postulated that captopril renography may be a suitable noninvasive tool to complement, or supplant, invasive RVRs as an index of renal perfusion and function in bilateral RVHT. Further studies in patients with RVHT appear warranted.

References

1 Nally JV, Clarke, HS, Grecos GP, et al: Effect of captopril on ^{99m}Tc-diethylenetriamine pentaacetic acid renograms in two-kidney, one-clip hypertension. Hypertension 1986;8:685–693.

2 Nally JV, Clarke HS, Gupta BK, et al: Captopril renography in two-kidney and one-kidney Goldblatt hypertension in dogs. J Nucl Med 1987;28:1171–1179.

3 Geyskes GG, Oei HY, Puylaert CBAJ, et al: Renovascular hypertension identified by captopril-induced changes in the renogram. Hypertension 1987;9:451–458.

Joseph V. Nally, Jr., MD, Department of Hypertension and Nephrology,
Desk A-101, The Cleveland Clinic Foundation, 9500 Euclid Avenue,
Cleveland, OH 44195–5042 (USA)

Blaufox MD, Hollenberg NK, Raynaud C (eds): Radionuclides in Nephro-Urology.
Contrib Nephrol. Basel, Karger, 1990, vol 79, pp 181–185

Detection of Renal Artery Stenosis by Means of Captopril Renography with ^{99m}Tc-DTPA

M. Dondi, M. Levorato, C. Corbelli, P. Zagni, A. Zuccalà, R. Gaggi, F. Marchetta, F. Losinno, A. Stella, M. Mirelli

Departments of Nuclear Medicine, Nephrology, Clinical Pharmacology, Radiology and Vascular Surgery, S. Orsola-Malpighi Policlinic Hospital, Bologna, Italy

An increasing number of patients is being referred for chronic dialysis for renal failure due to ischemic renal disease [1]. Renal artery stenosis (RAS) is therefore now being evaluated as a potential cause of renal function deterioration and not just as a cause of renovascular hypertension (RVH). Angiotensin-converting enzyme inhibition (ACEI) following captopril administration has already been proposed as a way of improving diagnostic accuracy of renal scintigraphy in the evaluation of hypertensive patients [2]. To date, most studies have dealt with RVH, diagnosed from blood pressure behavior after renal artery bypass graft or balloon angioplasty. However, renal artery revascularization, initially aimed at improving blood pressure levels, is now increasingly used for preserving renal function [3], potentially threatened by renovascular disease (RVD).

The aim of this study was to evaluate the role of captopril renography in detecting RAS in a population of patients referred for renal scan for hypertension, azotemia and/or reduced kidney size.

Materials and Methods

132 patients underwent conventional renal scintigraphy, followed within 72 h by a second study performed 1 h after oral administration of 50 mg of captopril. Abdominal aortography with selective renal angiography was obtained for all patients within 4 weeks. Of the 261 kidneys studied (3 patients had one kidney removed for reasons unrelated to hypertension), 168 were found to have no RAS, 25 RAS < 50% and 68 RAS > 50%.

Renal scintigraphy was performed with the patients imaged posteriorly, starting acquisition after intravenous injection of approximately 200 MBq of ^{99m}Tc-DTAP, collecting 1 frame every 10 s for a total of 1,120 s. Renograms were produced from a region of interest drawn around each kidney. Antihypertensive therapy was not withdrawn, except diuretics for at least 48 h and ACEI drugs for at least 7 days. Three parameters were employed to analyze scintigraphic studies: (a) split renal function (SRF), calculated as the relative tracer uptake of

Table 1. Population studied

	Kidneys (n = 261)	Patients (n = 132)
No RAS	168	65
RAS < 50%	25	15
RAS > 50%	68	52

each kidney divided by activity recorded over both kidneys from 90 to 150 s from injection: (b) tracer appearance into the pelvicalyceal system, and (c) upslope of the renogram. Parameters b and c were assessed from visual inspection of scintigraphic sequence and renograms.

To assess positivity of the provocative test with captopril, a decrease of at least 5% in SRF and/or a delay of time to maximum activity of more than 5 min together with a decrease in the upslope of the renogram, relative to baseline studies, were considered significant.

Results

For the purpose of this study, kidneys with no RAS were grouped together with those of RAS < 50% into group 1, while those kidneys supplied by an artery with RAS > 50% formed group 2 (table 1). An arterial lumen reduction of more than 50% was chosen as a limit beyond which RAS, other than being very likely the cause of RVH, is a potential threat to kidney function [3, 4]; it is for these reasons that patients with RAS > 50% are considered for revascularization at our institution.

Out of group 1, captopril renography correctly ruled out a RAS > 50% in all but 2 patients, 1 of which was bilaterally falsely positive. This patient, however, experienced a profound drop in blood pressure, with values below 90/60 mm Hg, probably because of a sodium-restricted diet. This study, repeated a few days later after sodium repletion, turned out correctly negative. In group 2, captopril renography did not show any change in seven kidneys supplied by an artery with a stenosis > 50%. Overall, unilateral RAS was identified both from an SFR reduction of more than 5% (fig. 1a) and from a delayed tracer appearance into the pelvicalyceal system (fig. 1b), though these two patterns did not necessarily appear together. Bilateral RAS characteristically showed a marked delay of time to maximum activity associated with a decrease of the upslope of the renogram (fig. 1c). Results in terms of sensitivity and specificity are reported in table 2.

Table 2. Results

	Kidneys	Patients
TP, n	61/68	48/52
TN, n	190/193	78/80
FP, n	3	2
FN, n	7	4
SENS, %	90	92
SPEC, %	98	97

n = Identification of patients with at least one renal artery with RAS > 50%.

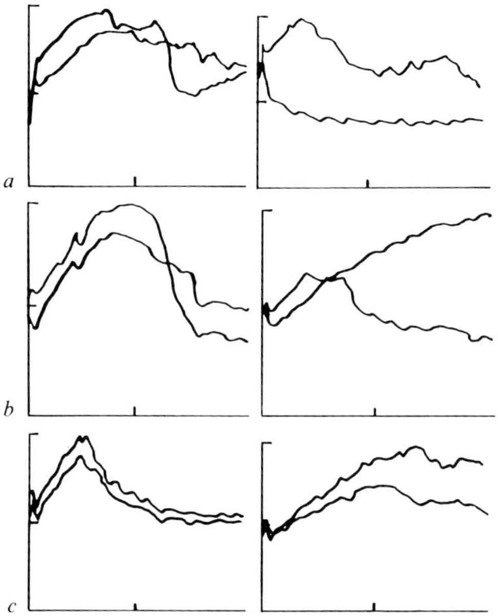

Fig. 1. Patterns of positive response to captopril administration: decrease of renal function from the side ipsilateral to RAS *(a)*; marked increase of time to peaking activity, either unilaterally *(b)* or bilaterally *(c)*.

Discussion

To date, renal scintigraphy after ACEI following captopril administration has been challenged as a means of identifying RVH, diagnosed by an improvement in blood pressure levels after renal artery revascularization [2].

There is however an increasing interest in the role of renal revascularization for the preservation of renal function [3]. Data support the hypothesis of progressive loss of functioning parenchyma, often with no exacerbation of hypertension [5], generally controllable by medical therapy [6–8]. Indeed, in many institutions, patients found to be affected by a RAS > 50% are considered for renal artery revascularization [8].

We feel therefore that captopril-enhanced renal scintigraphy, which proved to be such a promising tool in identifying RVH, should be tested as a means for detecting RAS > 50%, whether it be a source of hypertension or not. Two patterns of scintigraphic response to ACEI were identified: a marked decrease in glomerular filtration rate, expressed by a decrease in SRF from the side affected in unilateral RAS (fig. 1a) and a marked delay of time of maximum counts (fig. 1b). This second pattern, found to be typical of bilateral RAS (fig. 1c), might well reflect a less severe reduction in glomerular filtration associated with an increase in water reabsorption so that the tracer takes longer to move down the nephrons.

Our study demonstrated a high sensitivity of the test and an even higher specificity, providing a reliable means to rule out other causes of falsely positive results in conventional scintigraphy (nephrosclerosis, hypoplasia, obstructive uropathy, etc.). This latter parameter could have been better if the sodium intake of the patient with a bilaterally false-positive response had been monitored to avoid severe hypotension after ACEI.

In summary, captopril renography with ^{99m}Tc-DTPA improved specificity over conventional renal scintigraphy, a procedure burdened by a high false-positive rate which prevented its widespread application in the clinical setting. Moreover, stenoses < 50%, usually not considered for revascularization, never gave false-positive results, while sensitivity beyond that limit proved highly satisfactory. On the basis of our results we suggest captopril-enhanced renal scintigraphy as the first approach to patients referred for renal scan in their diagnostic work-up for RVD. If the provocative test turns out negative, it is reasonable to exclude RAS > 50%. Cases showing typical patterns of positivity can be referred for renal angiography. Only those cases with equivocal results will require a conventional renal scan for better evaluation of captopril-induced abnormalities.

References

1 Jacobson HR: Nephrology Forum. Ischemic renal disease: an overlooked clinical entity? Kidney Int 1988;34:729–743.

2 Oei HY, Geyskes GG, Roos GC, et al: Diagnosis of unilateral renal artery stenosis by captopril renography. Eur J Nucl Med 1984;9:A24.

3 Ying CY, Tifft CP, Gavras H, et al: Renal revascularization in the azotemic hypertensive patient resistant to therapy. N Engl J Med 1984;311:1070–1075.
4 Brawn LA, Ramsay LE: Is 'improvement' real with percutaneous transluminal angioplasty in the management of renovascular hypertension?. Lancet 1987;ii:1313–1316.
5 Dean RH, Kieffer RW, Smith BM, et al: Renovascular hypertension: anatomic and renal function changes during drug therapy. Arch Surg 1981;116:1408–1412.
6 Greninger P, Vetter H, Steurer J, et al: Captopril and kidney function in renovascular and essential hypertension. Nephron 1986;44 (suppl 1):91–95.
7 Blythe WB: Captopril and renal autoregulation. N Engl J Med 1983;308:390–391
8 Sicard GA, Etheridge EE, Maeser MN, et al: Improved renal function after renal artery revascularization. J Cardiovasc Surg 1985;26:157–161.

Dr. M. Dondi, Department of Nuclear Medicine, S. Orsola-Malpighi Policlinic Hospital, Via Albertoni 15, I–40138 Bologna (Italy)

Blaufox MD, Hollenberg NK, Raynaud C (eds): Radionuclides in Nephro-Urology.
Contrib Nephrol. Basel, Karger, 1990, vol 79, pp 186–189

The Measurement of Intrarenal Plasma Flow Distribution in Essential Hypertension

The Effect of Angiotensin-Converting Enzyme Inhibition

K.E. Britton, A.M. Al-Nahhas, C.C. Nimmon, M.J. Carroll, F. Fiore, K. Solanki, J. Bomanji

Department of Nuclear Medicine, St. Bartholomew's Hospital, West Smithfield, London, UK

The generally accepted features of established essential hypertension include a family history, a raised blood pressure associated with a normal cardiac output, a normal exchangeable sodium, a slightly reduced plasma volume [1] and a reduced plasma flow (RPF). Chasis and Redish [2] used *p*-aminohippurate clearance to show that renal plasma flow (F) in essential hypertension was reduced equally to each kidney. Given that the kidney has two populations of nephrons, the cortical and the juxtamedullary, with differing anatomical and physiological features, the question then is whether RPF is reduced to both populations to a similar extent, or just to the cortical nephrons (CN), or just to the juxtamedullary nephron (JMN).

Britton and Brown [3] showed that the intrarenal distribution of flow could be determined from the bimodal distribution of transit times of ^{131}I-orthoiodohippurate (OIH) through the kidney using probe renography. This approach was validated experimentally against microspheres by Wilkinson et al. [4] and adapted to the gamma camera by Gruenewald et al. [5] using ^{123}I-OIH. Since the administered amount of OIH is well below the tubular maximum, OIH is taken up by the proximal tubules of nephrons in proportion to their flow. CN have short loops of Henle with shorter transit times and JMN have long loops of Henle with longer transit times. As OIH is not reabsorbed from the tubular lumen, the population of OIH taking the shorter transit time through the renal parenchyme will be directly related to the proportion of flow to the CN. It was demonstrated that in essential hypertension, it was the reduction in flow to CN that accounted for the reduction of RPF in essential hypertension. Mean percentage CN flow was 84% of total flow in normotensive controls, but only 75% of total flow in essential hypertensive patients [5]. This data and the response of CN flow to treatment of the hypertensive patient with captopril lead Britton [6] to propose that essential hypertension was due to a disorder of CN control of autoregulation. The present study concerns the re-evaluation of this data through the use of a new angiotensin-converting enzyme inhibitor, Ramipril, in a placebo-controlled study of a small group of patients with essential hypertension.

Patient Protocol

Seven patients attending the authors' hypertension clinic with a family history of hypertensive disease were investigated conventionally to exclude renal, adrenal and other causes of hypertension. The protocol which had the approval of the District and Ethical Committee was explained to them and informed signed consent was obtained. The patient either received a placebo tablet or 10 mg Ramipril (both supplied by Hoechst Ltd UK) for 2–4 weeks, and then the alternative medication given. At the end of each period, blood pressure (BP) was monitored and renal function was measured as below.

Renal Function

The patient is well hydrated and then empties the bladder. The test is explained and the patient sits reclining with a computer-linked large field of view gamma camera (IGE-400AT) over the heart and kidney regions. The camera is set with a low-energy, general-purpose parallel-hole collimator and peaked for ^{123}I- or ^{99m}Tc as appropriate with a 20% window. A rapid intravenous injection of a measured amount, about 2 mCi (75 MBq) of ^{123}I-OIH or about 2.5 mCi (100 MBq) of ^{99m}Tc-MAG$_3$ (mercaptoacetyltriglycine) is given into the antecubital vein with the patient's arm abducted. Data collection continues for 20 min into a Varian V77 computer. Blood samples are taken 7, 17 and 44 min for the measurement of ERPF. ^{123}I-OIH is obtained from Amersham International and is free of ^{124}I. ^{99m}Tc-MAG$_3$ is obtained from Mallinckrodt Diagnostica, The Netherlands, and is prepared by the 'cold MAG$_3$' technique [7].

At the end of the study the data were displayed again and from the 2-min image regions of interest (ROI) for the left ventricle, the whole left and right kidneys and background regions were defined. To outline the pelvicalyceal area, a mean time image was constructed which is a functional image displaying the mean tracer time for each pixel, so that pixels with longer mean times will have higher image intensity, i.e., the pelvis and calyces. By excluding this high intensity area, the parenchymal area was defined and further divided into an outer zone, containing glomeruli that belong mainly to CN with few belonging to JMN, and an inner zone containing a mixture of both.

Using the activity time curve from the left ventricle ROI as the renal imput and curves from the outer zone and from the whole parenchyma, separate deconvolution analyses by the inverted matrix algorithm method were performed giving the activity retention in each zone. These impulse retention functions would result from a theoretical spike injection into the renal artery. The early vascular components were excluded and differentiation of these corrected retention functions gave the distribution of transit times through outer and the whole parenchymal zones.

A cross-correlation technique was used for noise reduction and the leading edge of the outer zone transit time distribution curve was fitted to the leading edge of the whole parenchymal zone distribution curve. Subtraction of the outer zone curve from the total

Table 1. Effect of Ramipril on intrarenal flow

	BP	CI	ERPF, ml/min	Cortical flow, ml/min
Placebo	172 ± 6 107 ± 6	1.44 ± 0.2	483 ± 20	207 ± 7
Ramipril	148 ± 10 90 ± 5	1.36 ± 0.1	564 ± 60	257 ± 21

parenchymal transit time distribution curve results in a new transit time distribution curve representing the transit of tracer through the JMN. On the assumption that CN in the inner zone have the same transit time distribution as those in the outer zone and different from those of JMN, the flow to the CN was obtained by comparing the heights of these CN and JMN transit time distribution curves and was presented as a percentage of the total flow for each kidney. The technique is given in more detail by Britton et al. [8] together with the methods for calculating the cardiac index (CI) and ERPF from the single injection of radiopharmaceutical. The relationship OIH = 1.5 MAG_3 + 40 ml/min was used [9] to determine ERPF when $^{99m}Tc-MAG_3$ was used and the results were normalised to the placebo CI to control for the effect of cardiac output on ERPF.

Results and Discussion

Both systolic and diastolic BP were significantly reduced by Ramipril (mean 172/107 to 148/90, $p = 0.05$). CI was not changed and the trend to an increase in ERPF was not significant. CN flow, however, increased from 207 ± 7 to 257 ± 21 ml/min ($p = 0.05$) (table 1).

This study has demonstrated that $^{99m}Tc-MAG_3$ is as good as ^{123}I-OIH for the measurement of the intrarenal flow distribution. Ramipril causes a significant increase in CN flow which at the same time gives a good reduction of blood pressure and confirms previous work with captopril [6]. This correction of a defect found in the kidneys of patients with essential hypertension, that of a reduced CN flow [5, 6], is relevant both to the aetiology and to the management of patients with essential hypertension [10].

References

1 Dickinson CJ: Neurogenic hypertension revisited. Clin Sci 1981;60:471–477.
2 Chasis H, Redish J: Effective renal blood flow in the separate kidneys of subjects with essential hypertension. J Clin Invest 1941;20:655–661.
3 Britton KE, Brown NJG: Clinical renography. London, Lloyd Luke, 1971.

4 Wilkinson SP, Bernard M, Pearce PC, et al: Validation of 'transit renography' for the determination of the intrarenal distribution of plasma flow: Comparison with the microsphere method in the anaesthetized rabbit and pig. Clin Sci Mol Med 1978;55:277–283.
5 Gruenewald SM, Nimmon CC, Nawaz MK, et al: A non-invasive gamma camera technique for the measurement of intrarenal flow distribution in man. Clin Sci 1981;61:385–389.
6 Britton KE: Essential hypertension: A disorder of cortical nephron control? Lancet 1981;ii:900–902.
7 Solanki KK, Al-Nahhas AM, Britton KE: 'Cold' $^{99m}Tc-MAG_3$; in Schmidt HAE, Burragi GL (eds): Nuclear Medicine. Proc Eur Nucl Med Congr, Milan 1988. Stuttgart, Schattauer, 1989, pp 443–446.
8 Britton KE, Nawaz MK, Nimmon CC, et al: Total and intrarenal flow distribution in healthy subjects: Technique, acute effects of Ibopamine and of Indoramin. Nephron 1986;43:265–273.
9 Britton KE, Jafri RA, Nimmon CC: Comparison of the clearance of technetium-99m MAG_3 and iodine-131 OIH. J Nucl Med 1988;29:1878–1879.
10 Britton KE: Radioisotope renal function studies in essential hypertension. Cardiology 1985;72(suppl 1):22–29.

K.E. Britton, MD, Department of Nuclear Medicine, St. Bartholomew's Hospital, West Smithfield, GB–London EC1A 7BE (UK)

Blaufox MD, Hollenberg NK, Raynaud C (eds): Radionuclides in Nephro-Urology.
Contrib Nephrol. Basel, Karger, 1990, vol 79, pp 190–195

Captopril Renography and Duplex Sonography: Comparison of Two Noninvasive Methods for the Diagnosis and Follow-Up in Renovascular Hypertension

K. Kletter, G. Mostbeck, R. Dudczak
First Medical Department, University of Vienna, Austria

The prevalence of renovascular hypertension (RVH) in hypertensive patients is low. However, due to the recent advances in percutaneous transluminal angioplasty (PTA) and the better prognosis for patients with repair of the stenosis compared to patients treated by antihypertensive drugs alone, there has been a renewed interest in screening for potentially correctable RVH [1, 2]. Since there are no pathognomonic clinical characteristics for RVH allowing a better selection of patients for further investigations [1], a screening test for RVH has to be noninvasive. Conventional radioisotope renography and intravenous urography both failed to achieve a suitable sensitivity and specificity in this question [1, 2]. Digital subtraction angiography (DAS) is considered the screening test of choice for renal artery stenosis (RAS), yet the rate of uninterpretable results is higher if the contrast media is injected into a peripheral vein. Therefore, the arterial injection of the contrast media is required, but this invalidates the noninvasive nature of the method. In addition, DSA lacks functional information to achieve a sufficient high likelihood for potentially correctable RVH by PTA [6]. From recent reports it appears that captopril renography (CRG) will greatly improve the efficacy of radionuclide studies in the diagnosis and prognosis of RVH [3–6]. CRG may even be advantageous over renal vein plasma renin concentration (PRC) determinations and the plasma renin captopril test [5, 6]. A further noninvasive test for the detection of RAS is duplex sonography (DS). This method was applied by Greene et al. [7] for the noninvasive measurement of renal artery blood flow. DS has shown a surprisingly high sensitivity and specificity for RVH in the hand of some authors [8] and was proposed as a screening tool by several groups [8, 9].

The aim of our retrospective study was to compare the potential for CRG and DS for diagnosing RVH in patients with known RAS.

Patients and Methods

Twenty-four patients with angiographically documented RAS were studied. In addition, PRC was determined before and after captopril by a radioimmunoassay. Eight patients had bilateral stenoses; out of the remaining 16 patients with unilateral stenosis, 2 had a solitary kidney. The cause of the stenosis was fibromuscular hyperplasia in 7 and atherosclerosis in 17 patients. PTA was performed in 16 patients, in 2 patients PTA was done on both sides. Following PTA, 14 patients were controlled by CRG and 9 by DS.

Renography

Baseline and captopril renograms were obtained in all patients. Antihypertensives and diuretics were withdrawn at least 48 h prior to the studies. Forty-five minutes before renography, 10 ml/kg b.w. fluid and during CRG, 25 mg captopril were administered. ^{123}I-OIH renography (15 min) was performed first followed by ^{99m}Tc-DTPA renography (7 min). The criteria for the evidence of a hemodynamically significant RAS were derived from results obtained from patients with essential hypertension [6] and were defined as follows: a delay in peak activity (T_{max}) in the CRG exceeding 2 min as compared with the baseline value and/or a lower uptake of ^{99m}Tc-DTPA in comparison with the uptake of ^{123}I-OIH after captopril (uptake quotient ^{123}I-OIH/^{99m}Tc-DTPA > 1.2).

Duplex Sonography

DS examinations were performed on fasted patients in the supine position during light inspiration. A real-time sector scanner (3.5–7.5 MHz transducers) with a pulsed Doppler probe operating at a frequency of 3 or 5 MHz was used. The sample volume of the Doppler probe was adapted to the diameter of the renal arteries (RA) and ranged from 1.5 × 1.5 to 5 × 5 mm. A Doppler filter of 100 Hz was used for smoothing. RA were scanned longitudinally in transverse abdominal planes. Care was taken to evaluate the RA from the origin of the aorta up to the renal hilum. The sample volume cursor was placed to the center of the vessel volume. The relative angle between the Doppler beam axis and the longitudinal axis of the RA was adjusted within the range of 30–60°. After fast Fourier analysis the Doppler spectra were displayed together with real-time images; data were documented on X-ray film (fig. 1). The criteria for the evidence of a hemodynamically significant RAS by DS were as follows: A peak systolic frequency shift of more than 4 MHz according to the acceleration of the blood flow on the site of the stenosis and a spectral broadening of the Doppler wave form corresponding to a turbulent flow [9].

Results

Due to anatomical variations, visualization of the RA from the aortic origin up to the renal hilum by DS was only partly possible. Accordingly, DS results were arranged into three groups: (a) good visualization (b) partial visualization (DS investigation of RA possible only near aortic origin or at the renal hilum and (c) no visualization. For the 23 right RA investigated, visualization was good in 12 (52%) and partial in 5 (22%); 6 RA were not visualized. Results for the left RA (n = 23) were poorer;

a b c d

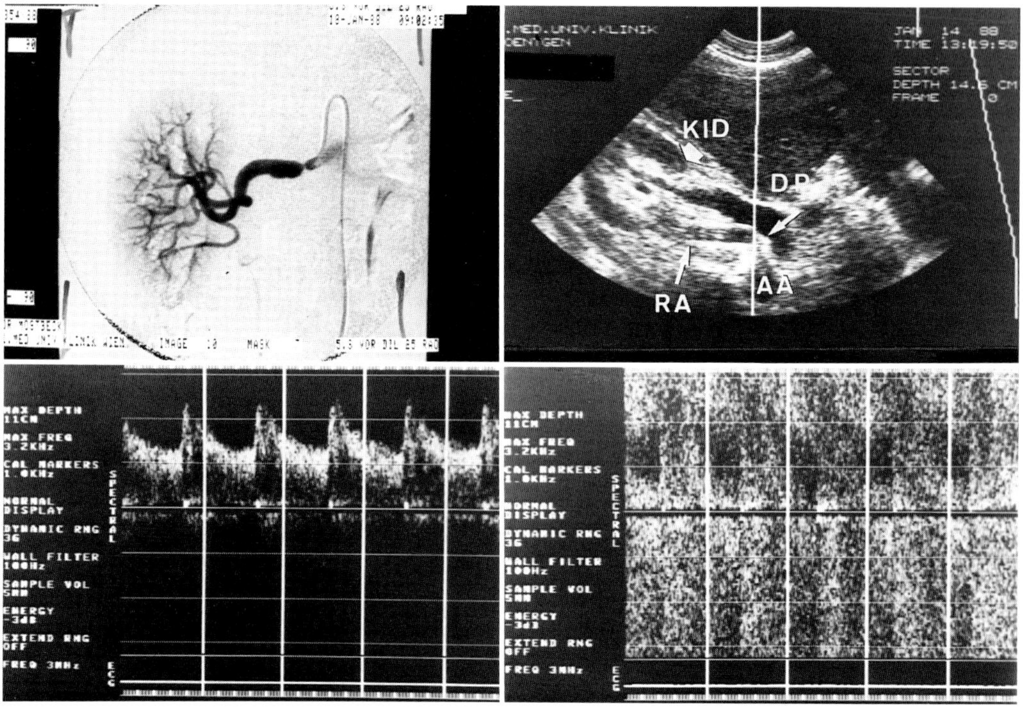

Fig. 1. a Angiographic image of a patient with a 90% stenosis of the right RA. *b* Real-time image showing the right kidney (KID), the right RA (RA) with the Doppler cursor (DP) and the abdominal aorta (AA). *c* Normal Doppler spectrum before the site of the stenosis. *d* Doppler spectrum at the site of the stenosis demonstrating frequency shift and spectral broadening.

visualization was good only in 5 (22%), partial in 10 (43%) and no visualization was obtained in 8 RA.

The sensitivity for the detection of RAS by DS and CRG in relation to the angiographically determined degree of the stenosis is given in table 1. The results show a distinct improvement for the sensitivity for both methods with higher graded RAS. However, due to the high number of technically inadequate results the figures for DS are only approximate. Taking into account only DS results with good visualization of RA, a stenosis with a degree ⩾90% was always detected.

In 2 patients with only minimal residual kidney function on the side of the stenosis, no statement on the functional significance was possible by CRG. DS as well as CRG was false-positive in 1 patient (no stenosis detected by angiography).

Table 1. Sensitivity for the detection of RAS by CRG and DS in relation to the grade of the stenosis

Grade of stenosis	Number of vessels	Positive CRG		Positive DS	
		n	%	n	%
≥ 90%	17	12	71	8	47
> 50% < 90%	11	4	36	2	18
≤ 50%	4	1	25	1	25

Table 2. Correctness of DS and CRG for the diagnosis RVH in 16 patients: results were validated by blood pressure behavior after PTA

Investigation	True-positive	True-negative	False-positive	False-negative
DS[1]	7	1	1	3
CRG	12	3	0	1

[1] RA were not visualized in 4 patients.

The results of the plasma renin captopril test (PRC-CT) were classified as follows: (A) no or only minimal increase after ACE inhibition (< 1 GU (Goldblatt unit) $\times 10^{-4}$/ml); (B) increase in PRC between > 1 and < 3 GU $\times 10^{-4}$/ml, and (C) increase in PRC > 3GU $\times 10^{-4}$/ml (overshooting renin secretion corresponding to a positive captopril test). Accordingly, 9, 8 and 7 patients belonged to groups A, B and C respectively. In all patients of group C the CRG was positive. DS showed good or partial visualization of RA in 5 and was positive in 3 patients of this group. CRG was positive in 5 patients of group B ($n = 8$) and in 5 patients of group A ($n = 9$). The corresponding results for DS in patients with good or partial visualization of the RA were 4 for group B ($n = 5$) and 3 for group A ($n = 7$).

The results of DS and CRG for the evidence of RVH were validated by the blood pressure changes after PTA in 16 patients (table 2). DS control studies in 9 patients after PTA excluded correctly a residual stenosis or a restenosis, noteworthy DS was true-negative in 1 patient where CRG suggested a restenosis. CRG studies became normal in patients with blood pressure normalization except in 1 patient. CRG remained unchanged (normal in respect to RVH) in patients who did not improve in blood pressure after PTA.

Discussion

DS would appear to be the ideal noninvasive screening test for patients with a low prevalence for a disease with regard to the invasiveness. In contrast to CRG, no injection or drug administration is necessary, therefore side effects cannot occur. DS has no concomitant radiation burden. However, there are some substantial disadvantages of DS, e.g. results are strongly dependent on patient characteristics and operator skill. But even if performed by an experienced investigator many technically inadequate studies result. Thus, because of the high rate of poor visualization of the RA, in contrast to other authors [8, 9], we cannot recommend DS as a screening test for RVH. In agreement with the previous studies we found a high sensitivity for the detection of RAS by DS in case of good visualization of the RA and a high grade of the stenosis. The rate of false-positive results for DS can be expected to be low.

CRG predicted correctly the functional significance of a stenosis (except in 1 case) as validated by the blood pressure behavior after repair of the stenosis. CRG lacks another shortcoming of DS, that is the failure to detect a stenosis located behind the main RA. In accordance with our previous studies [5, 6], CRG was superior to the PRC-CT. Difficulties in the interpretation of the CRG result from kidneys with strongly reduced function. DS may establish or exclude RVH in these cases. In addition it should be mentioned that ultrasonography of the kidneys may yield useful morphological information, e.g. the evidence of hydronephrosis, and thus facilitate the interpretation of CRG results.

In conclusion, CRG is preferable to DS in the diagnosis of RVH; in case of good visualization of the RA, DS may be used for follow-up after PTA and may substitute CRG in special cases.

References

1 Carmichael DS, Mathias CJ, Snell ME: Detection and investigation of renal artery stenosis. Lancet 1982;i:667–670.

2 Havey RJ, Krumlovsky F, del Greco F, et al: Screening for renovascular hypertension. Is renal digital subtraction angiography the preferred noninvasive test? Jama 1985;245:388–393.

3 Fommei E, Ghione S, Palla L, et al: Renal scintigraphic captopril test in the diagnosis of renovascular hypertension. Hypertension 1987;10:212–220.

4 Sfakianakis GN, Bourgoignie JJ, Jaffe D, et al: Single-dose captopril scintigraphy in the diagnosis of renovascular hypertension. J Nucl Med 1987;28:1383–1392.

5 Kletter K, Leitha T, Dudczak R: Captopril renography and captopril test in unilateral and bilateral renal artery stenosis. J Nucl Med 1988;29:850.

6 Kletter K: New trends in radioisotope function studies. Improved diagnostic potential by pharmacological intervention and by quantitative analysis. Wien Klin Wocheschr 1988;100(suppl. 177).
7 Greene ER, Venters MD, Avasthi PS et al: Noninvasive characterization of renal artery blood flow. Kidney Int 1981;20:523–529.
8 Ferretti G, Salomone A, Castagno PL, et al: Renovascular hypertension: a noninvasive duplex scanning screening. Int Angiol 1988;7:219–223.
9 Robertson R, Murphy A, Dubbins PA: Renal artery stenosis: the use of duplex ultrasound as a screening technique. Br J Radiol 1988;61:196–201.

K. Kletter, MD, PhD, First Medical Department, University of Vienna, Lazarettgasse 14, A–1090 Vienna (Austria)

Blaufox MD, Hollenberg NK, Raynaud C (eds): Radionuclides in Nephro-Urology.
Contrib Nephrol. Basel, Karger, 1990, vol 79, pp 196–199

Results of Quantification of Frusemide Response in ^{123}I-Hippuran Renal Studies of Unilateral Renal Artery Stenosis

F. Flueckiger, G.F. Fueger, K. Hausegger, R. Nicoletti

Department of Radiology, Division of Nuclear Medicine, Graz, Austria

Renal radionuclide studies (RRS) are well established in the assessment of renal ischemia among hypertensive patients. The quantification of static and dynamic RRS helps to increase their specificity and to assess the extent of diminution of renal function in RAS. In addition to the 'dynamic' parameters of relative unilateral clearance, transit time, and time to peak, we calculate in all RRS (not only in urinary tract obstruction) the frusemide response (FR) and a retention index (RI) as further parameters of renal (i.e. tubular) function. The present study was designed to reveal possible differences in the degree of FR and RI between essential (EH) and renovascular hypertension (RVH).

Methods

We studied three groups of patients: 50 patients without renal disease and without hypertension (normal reference group); 23 patients with EH, yet without RAS, and 57 patients with RVH due to hemodynamically significant unilateral renal artery stenosis (HSRAS). Eleven patients with HSRAS underwent successful percutaneous transluminal angioplasty (PTA) and were reexamined 2–6 weeks after intervention. Patients with renal parenchymal disease, tumor, cysts, renal insufficiency, urinary tract obstruction, nephroptosis or diabetes were excluded from the study. After hydration the dynamic RRS was performed from posterior with the patient sitting. Computer acquisition was started after intravenous injection of 10 μCi/kg b.w. ^{123}I-hippuran. The data from the scintillation camera were acquired in frame mode in a 64×64 matrix: 30 frames of 10 s each and 10 frames of 1 min, further 10 frames of 1 min after intravenous injection of 40 mg frusemide. Computer processing of the data was performed automatically, with manual correction of the ROIs if necessary. The FR for each kidney was assessed by the difference in renal tracer content before and 10 min after injection. The activity before (Ab) and the activity after (Aa) was expressed as percentage of peak renal activity. The frusemide-induced washout of activity from the renal parenchyma was quantified as a percentage of the Ab (fig. 1). The renal tracer content before and 10 min after frusemide injection is the basis for the RI (fig. 1).

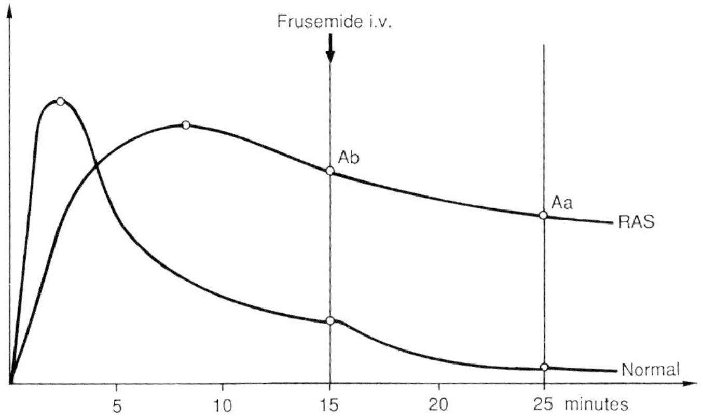

$$FR = \frac{(Ab\text{-}Aa) \times 100}{Ab} \qquad RI = \frac{Ab \times Aa}{10}$$

Fig. 1. Mode of the calculation of frusemide response and retention index.

Table 1. Values of frusemide response and retention index obtained for the three groups

	n	Frusemide response, %	Retention index
Normal	50	> 50	< 20
Essential hypertension	23	70 ± 25	12 ± 7
Renovascular hypertension	57	22 ± 7	410 ± 210

Results

The values of the FR and RI obtained in the three groups are presented in table 1. In EH the two parameters do not differ from the normal range whereas in RVH in the poststenotic kidney the FR was diminished and the RI elevated significantly. The values of FR and RI before and after PTA in the 11 treated patients are presented in figure 2. The ranges of the parameters correlated well with the arteriography and the blood pressure.

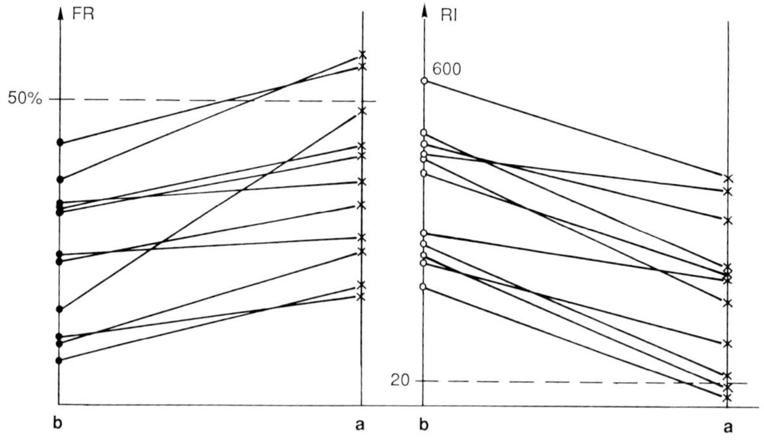

Fig. 2. FR and RI in the 11 PTA-treated patients at the side of the RAS before (b) and after (a) treatment.

Discussion

In healthy kidneys, frusemide increases the renal blood flow and the glomerular filtration. The effectiveness of frusemide is caused by inhibition of the tubular reabsorption of sodium and possibly by inhibition of the tubuloglomerular feedback (supposed by Thurau [3]) but necessitates that frusemide is available in the distal tubular lumen and this in turn depends on the proximal tubular anion transport mechanism. That transport mechanism is disturbed in several renal diseases, for example in renal ischemia [3]. The most important prerequisite for the effectiveness of frusemide is the maintenance of a high glomerular filtration rate.

RVH caused by RAS leads to a stimulation of the renin-angiotensin-aldosterone system. The consequence of renal ischemia is an excessive reabsorption of sodium and water. This fact leads to parenchymal tracer retention (elevated RI), which is the basis of an abnormal renogram in RVH [1].

In a poststenotic kidney the FR is relatively lower than in the normal because of reduced basic renal blood flow and glomerular filtrate and the disturbed proximal tubular anion transport mechanism. Furthermore, frusemide in HSRAS leads to an additional stimulation of the renin-angiotensin-aldosterone system followed by further diminution of the blood flow. Such a reduced FR was observed in patients with RAS on sonography and intravenous urography: the increase in renal size after intravenous injection of frusemide was less in ischemic than in healthy kidneys [2–4]. We quantified FR and RI to assess this diminished washout of tracer content. Our results show that the FR is diminished and the RI is elevated in HSRAS and that the parameters correlate well with the degree of stenosis before and after PTA. We believe that frusemide intervention and quantification of RRS represents important steps in the detection of renal ischemia as well as in the assessment of renal function in a poststenotic kidney.

References

1 Freeman LM, Johnson PM: Clinical Scintillation Imaging. New York, Grune & Stratton, 1975, pp 376–382.
2 Maggiore Q, Curatola G, Zoccali C: Effect of furosemide on renal size: Ultrasonic characterization of renovascular hypertension. Nephron 1982;31:45–50.
3 Thurau K: Kontrolle des Glomerulumfiltrats durch den tubuloglomerulären Rückkoppelungsmechanismus und seine Beeinflussung durch Furosemid. Nieren- und Hochdruckkrankheiten 1985;6:221–223.
4 Wolf GL: Rationale and use of vasodilated excretory urogram in screening for renovascular hypertension. Am J Roentgenol 1973;119:692–700

Dr. Fritz Flueckiger, Department of Radiology, Auenbruggerplatz 9, LKH,
A–8036 Graz (Austria)

Blaufox MD, Hollenberg NK, Raynaud C (eds): Radionuclides in Nephro-Urology.
Contrib Nephrol. Basel, Karger, 1990, vol 79, pp 200–204

Usefulness of Renal Sequential Scintigraphy for the Evaluation of Antihypertensive Drugs

G. La Cava [a], *R. Sciagrà* [a], *L. Scarti* [b], *L. Poggesi* [b], *G. Masotti* [b], *U. Meldolesi* [a]

[a] Department of Clinical Pathophysiology, Nuclear Medicine, and [b] Clinica Medica I, University of Florence, Italy

In essential hypertension a reduction of renal blood flow, due to an overautoregulation of the cortical nephrons, has been postulated as a possible causative mechanism [1]. Antihypertensive drugs which increase renal blood flow could be beneficial in interrupting this hypertensive process. On the contrary, drugs like most β-blockers or thiazide diuretics, which directly or indirectly reduce renal blood flow, will in the long term be less effective and probably harmful [1]. It seems therefore reasonable to test the renal effects of antihypertensive drugs possibly using a reproducible method for estimating kidney function like renal sequential scintigraphy (RSS).

Methods

Two different antihypertensive drugs were evaluated: intravenously infused clonidine for the therapy of severe hypertension and hypertensive emergencies, and oral indenolol, a noncardioselective β-blocker with intrinsic sympathomimetic activity, proposed for the long-term treatment of moderate hypertension. Two different patient populations were therefore examined. The first (group A) included 13 patients (5 males and 8 females, age range 36–60 years) affected by severe hypertension (diastolic pressure > 130 mm Hg), resistant to the previously used antihypertensive drugs and who were evaluated in order to find an effective treatment. The second (group B) was composed of 12 subjects (8 males and 4 females, age range 37–68 years) affected by WHO grades I–II hypertension, who were evaluated for establishing a well-tolerated long-term antihypertensive therapy. In both groups hypertension could be defined as essential after an accurate clinical and instrumental evaluation. Informed consent was obtained from each patient.

After a washout period (5 days for group A and 4 weeks for B) all patients underwent a baseline RSS. Three days later, group A patients were intravenously infused with clonidine (Catapres®, Boehringer Ingelheim) at a rate of 15 μg/min, and group B subjects received an oral dose of 120 mg indenolol (Securpres®, Poli Company). A second RSS was then performed in group A, after having reached a significant decrease (< 105 mm Hg) of the mean arterial

Table 1. ^{131}I-hippuran renal transit times

Transit times (sec)	Group A		Group B	
	baseline	clonidine	baseline	indenolol
Minimum PTT	128 ± 35	146 ± 44	165 ± 40	158 ± 27
Mean PTT	227 ± 75**	289 ± 100	298 ± 44	274 ± 56
Minimum GTT	147 ± 41	166 ± 53	205 ± 40	191 ± 43
Mean GTT	322 ± 88*	370 ± 146	366 ± 70	355 ± 97

PTT = Parenchymal transit time; GTT = global transit time.
*$p < 0.001$; **$p < 0.0005$.

pressure (MAP: diastolic pressure plus one third of the pulse pressure) and in group B 2 h after drug administration, when according to previous studies the maximal antihypertensive effect is usually achieved [2].

RSS was performed with the patient lying supine, using a large field of view gamma camera (ZLC, Siemens) equipped with a medium-energy collimator and interfaced with a Hewlett-Packard A900 computer. A dose of 222 kBq/kg body weight of ^{131}I-hippuran was injected for the measurement of the effective renal plasma flow (ERPF) and a 28-min acquisition was performed. The data were acquired in list mode with a 5 s resolution on a 64 × 64 matrix. Using our described procedure the single kidney ERPF was calculated [3, 4]. Renal vascular resistance (RVR) was calculated as the ratio of MAP and renal blood flow and was converted from mm Hg/l/min into dyn s cm^{-5} by multiplying by 80. The renal global and parenchymal transit times of ^{131}I-hippuran were also measured [5].

Results

The MAP decreased significantly with both treatments: in group A from 156.5 ± 15 to 103 ± 11 ($p < 0.0001$) and in group B from 119.1 ± 8 to 99.1 ± 11 ($p < 0.0001$) (fig. 1).

In group A the single kidney ERPF was significantly increased from a baseline value of 175 ± 52 to 221 ± 72 ml min^{-1} ($p < 0.001$). Simultaneously a significant reduction of the RVR was achieved: from a baseline value of 20,787 ± 8,029 to 10,945 ± 5,107 dyn s cm^{-5} ($p < 0.001$) (fig. 1a). Finally a significant increase of both the mean global and parenchymal transit times could be demonstrated (table 1).

In group B the single kidney ERPF increased from a baseline value of 222 ± 71 to 248 ± 69 ml min^{-1} ($p < 0.01$), whereas there was a decrease of the RVR from 12,946 ± 4,556 to 9,157 ± 2,083 dyn s cm^{-5} ($p < 0.002$)

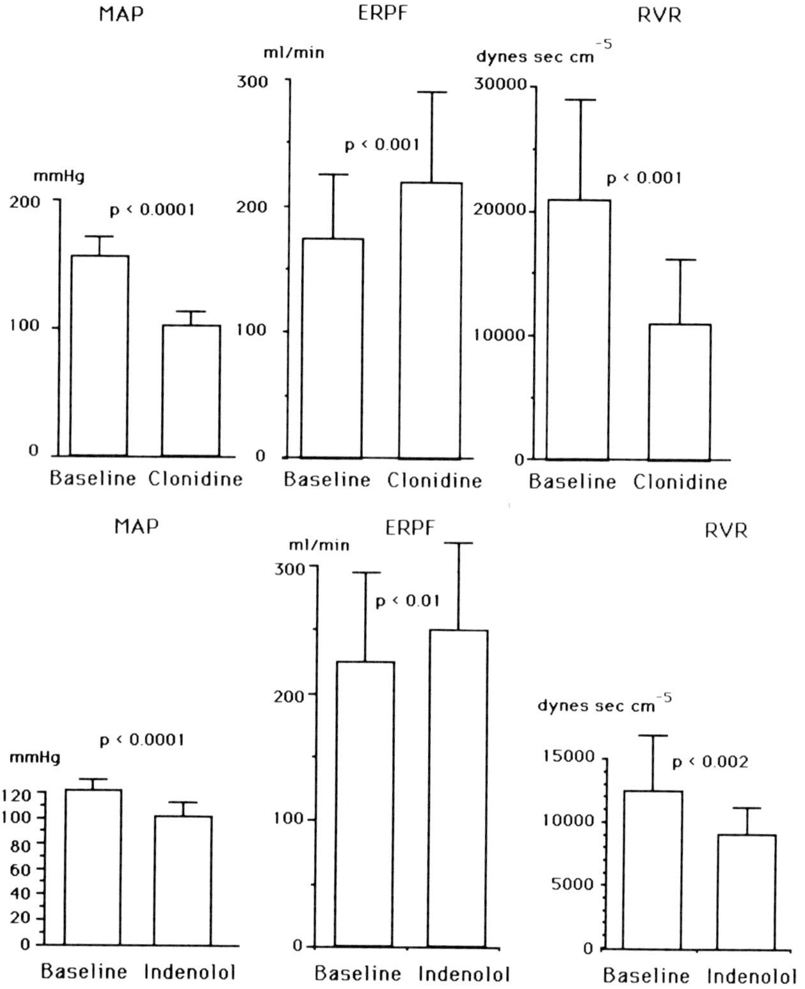

Fig. 1. *a* MAP (left), ERPF (middle) and RVR (right) under baseline conditions and after clonidine infusion in the patients of group A. *b* MAP (left), ERPF (middle) and RVR (right) under baseline conditions and after oral administration of indenolol in the patients of group B.

(fig. 1b). In group B no changes in either global or parenchymal transit times could be found (table 1).

Noteworthy adverse reactions were not registered. In group A slight somnolence and mouth dryness were reported by some patients; furthermore, in all of them atonia of the pelvis could be observed in the scintigraphic images.

Discussion

The absence of adverse effects on renal hemodynamics is certainly a main point in the evaluation of antihypertensive drugs. This problem deserves an accurate assessment and methods which allow the measurement of the single kidney function in a reproducible way should be preferred. Our preliminary experience had already demonstrated the accuracy and reproducibility of our approach for the estimate of renal function using sequential scintigraphy with external measurements only [3, 4].

The results of this study confirm that the intravenous infusion of clonidine can be safely and effectively employed to treat severe hypertension and hypertensive emergencies. In this acute setting the absence of a reduction in renal blood flow is highly desirable, since the renal function is often already impaired in these patients, as demonstrated by the low ERPF baseline values in our group A. The changes in renal transit times can be explained: the increase in the global transit times could be attributed to the stagnation of urine in the atonic pelvis, whereas the increase of the parenchymal transit times could be justified by a relatively greater vasodilating effect on the efferent arteriole and with an ensuing fall in the filtration pressure. An acute inhibition of the renin-angiotensin system, also highly desirable in hypertensive emergencies, could be the cause of this phenomenon [6, 7].

The problem of renal blood flow reduction is also a relevant drawback of antihypertensive therapy with most β-blockers. Of them only nadolol, because of direct vasodilatory action on renal vasculature, and those with high intrinsic sympathomimetic activity, such as pindolol, seem devoid of this effect [1]. Previous experiences with indenolol suggested its intrinsic sympathomimetic activity and demonstrated a reduction of peripheral vascular resistance [2, 8], which seems to be maintained also after prolonged treatment [8]. The results of our study show for the first time a favorable effect of indenolol even on renal hemodynamics, at least after acute administration. Further studies, for which RSS seeems the ideal tool, are needed in order to assess the changes induced on renal function by long-term therapy with this agent.

References

1 Britton KE: Radioisotopic renal function studies in essential hypertension. Cardiology 1985;72(suppl 1):22–29.
2 Poggesi L, Masotti G, Boddi M, et al: Effects of indenolol on blood pressure, lower limb blood flow adrenergic reflexes, and plasma renin activity. Clin Pharmacol Ther 1987;41:345–350.

3 Formiconi AR, La Cava G, Morotti A, et al: Renal sequential scintigraphy: unilateral clearance rate determination based on external measurements only. Eur J Nucl Med 1983;8:150–154.
4 La Cava G, Sciagrà R, Formiconi AR, et al: Validation of a new method for quantifying renal function; in Blaufox MD, Hollenberg NK, Raynaud C (eds): Radionuclides in Nephro-Urology. Contrib Nephrol, Basel, Karger, 1990, vol 79, pp. 82–86.
5 Britton KE: Advances in dynamic renal imaging; in Medical Radionuclide Imaging. IAEA, Vienna 1981. vol 2, pp 341–350.
6 Weber MA, Case DB, Baer L, et al: Renin and aldosterone suppression in the antihypertensive action of clonidine. Am J Cardiol 1976;38:825–830.
7 Pettinger WA, Keeton TK, Campbell WB, et al: Evidence for a renal alpha-adrenergic receptor inhibiting renin release. Circ Res 1976;38:338–346.
8 Malacco E, Mailland F, Bosisio E, et al: Acute and long-term haemodynamic effects of propanolol and indenolol in hypertension. Eur J Clin Pharmacol 1986;30:157–160.

Giuseppe La Cava, MD, Department of Clinical Pathophysiology,
Nuclear Medicine, University of Florence, Viale Morgagni 85,
I–50134 Florence (Italy)

Special Reports on Collaborative Studies in Captopril Renography

Blaufox MD, Hollenberg NK, Raynaud C (eds): Radionuclides in Nephro-Urology. Contrib Nephrol. Basel, Karger, 1990, vol 79, pp 205–210

Captopril Radionuclide Test in Renovascular Hypertension

A European Multicenter Study[1]

E. Fommei, L. Mezzasalma, S. Ghione

CNR Institute of Clinical Physiology, Pisa, Italy

The anatomical cause of renovascular hypertension resides in an obstruction of the renal blood flow (usually by a renal artery stenosis either by fibrodysplasia or by atherosclerosis). Its pathophysiological mechanism is sustained by the activation of the pressor renin-angiotensin-aldosterone system.Therefore, its diagnostic workup requires both anatomical and functional investigations, which comprehend costly and invasive procedures such as renal arteriography and bilateral renal vein catheterization with sampling for plasma renin activity [1, 2].

[1] *Participants of the Multicenter Study:* Dr. R.P. Baum, Department of Nuclear Medicine, University Hospital, Frankfurt am Main; Dr. I. Beuerlein, Nuklear-medizin, Allgemeines Krankenhaus Harburg, Hamburg, FRG; Dr. E. Brianzoni, Servizio di Medicina Nucleare, Ospedale di Macerata, Macerata; Dr. M. Dondi, Servizio di Medicina Nucleare, Ospedale S. Orsola Malpighi, Bologna, Italy; Dr. E. Fommei, Hypertension Unit, Institute of Clinical Physiology, Pisa, Italy; Dr. M. Fraile, Servicio de Medicina Nuclear, Hosp. General 'Vall d'Hebron', Barcelona, Spain; Dr. D. Granjon, Service de Medicine Nucleaire, Hopital Nord CHRU, Saint Priest en Jarez, France; Dr. R. Hoschl, Department of Nuclear Medicine, Royal North Shore Hospital, St. Leonards, Australia; Dr. G. Jensen, Department of Nephrology, Sahlgrenska Sjnkhuset, Göteborg, Sweden; Prof. P. Jezersek, Univerzitetna Interna Klinika, Ljubljana, Yugoslavia; Dr. E. Länsimies, Department of Clinical Physiology, University Central Hospital, Kuopio, Finland; Dr. R. Müller-Suur, Department of Clinical Physiology, Danderyds Hospital, Danderyd, Sweden; Dr. G.A. van Montfrans, Academic Medical Center, Amsterdam; Dr. H.Y. Oei, Department of Nuclear Medicine, Academisch Ziekenhuis, Rotterdam, The Netherlands; Dr. A. Piepsz, Service des Radioisotopes, Hôpital Universitaire St. Pierre, Brussels, Belgium; Dr. M. Poropat, Department of Nuclear Medicine, University Hospital, Zagreb, Yugoslavia; Dr. C.G. Santos, Servicio de Medicina Nuclear, Hospital de Clinicas de P. Alegre, Porto Alegre, Brasil; Dr. J.C. Wautrecht, Chirurgie Vasculaire, Hôpital Universitaire Erasme, Brussels, Belgium;

Executive Committee: Dr. E. Fommei, Pisa, Italy; Dr. S. Ghione, Pisa, Italy: Dr. I. Gordon, London, UK; Dr. A.J.W. Hilson, London, UK; Dr. H.Y. Oei, Rotterdam, The Netherlands; Dr. A. Piepsz, Brussels, Belgium.

Recently, the captopril radionuclide test (CRT) (captopril renography, renal scintigraphy under ACE inhibition, etc.) has gained widespread interest as a promising noninvasive diagnostic tool for renovascular hypertension, since it explores an intrarenal aspect which may be specifically associated with renal hypoperfusion, i.e. the dependence of glomerular filtration rate on angiotensin II activation. In fact, by comparison of post-captopril with baseline data, this scintigraphic test allows the detection of the decrease of glomerular filtration rate that may be induced by angiotensin II inhibition in kidneys ipsilateral to arterial stenoses. By yielding both morphological and functional renal information the test may be particularly useful for the diagnosis of functionally significant renal hypoperfusion, as reported by a growing number of scientific papers in recent years [3–10]. Either glomerular filtration markers (e.g. ^{99m}Tc-DTPA) [3–7, 10] or tubular secretion markers (e.g. hippuran or MAG_3) [4–6, 8, 9] were used to this purpose. For the former tracers a positive response to captopril is represented by a decrease or suppression of uptake, for the latter by a delay of excretion.

Although renovascular hypertension is considered to be the most common secondary form of arterial hypertension, its incidence in an individual center involved in the diagnosis and treatment of arterial hypertension is relatively low. For this reason the evaluation of the clinical usefulness of a test devised for the diagnosis of this disease would be greatly facilitated by a collaborative study of various centers.

Historical Background

The idea to initiate a collaborative study on CRT started at the European Meeting of Nuclear Medicine in London (September 1985). During the International Symposium 'Radionuclides in Nephro-Urology' held in Lausanne (May 1986) a preliminary protocol was developed by several experts and tested in a pilot study by E. Dubovski, University of Alabama, Birmingham (USA), J. Nally, Medical College of Ohio, Toledo (USA) and M. Aurell, University of Göteborg (Sweden). The data were received by the Hypertension Unit of the Institute of Clinical Physiology, Pisa (Italy). The final protocol was written during a workshop held in Pisa (April 1987).

General Design of the Protocol

Two contrasting needs were soon recognized: standardization and practicability. Optimally, this kind of study would have to be performed:

(1) in a series of patients representative of the general hypertensive population; (2) with a uniform patient selection in all centers; and (3) with adherence to a single fully standardized protocol as concerned radioisotope methodology, strategies of diagnostic workup for renovascular hypertension and criteria for intervention. However, it was understood that in most centers the prevailing population would have consisted of referred patients suspected to have renovascular hypertension and only few centers would have been able (willing) to systematically evaluate nonselected hypertensive patients and to adhere to a fully standardized diagnostic and therapeutic protocol. Further aspects to be taken into account were: (1) the lack of a financial support: each center had to carry out its own part at its own expense; (2) the central role of the Nuclear Medicine Departments; and (3) the lack of any a priori knowledge of a method of choice. Therefore, it was decided to pursue a more practical, clinically-oriented approach, i.e. to obtain a picture on how CRT works in various different clinical settings.

Description of the Procotol

Selection of Patients

Eligible for this study were defined hypertensive patients who, on the basis of the clinical judgement of the referring physician, would benefit from a diagnostic evaluation which included renal angiography and CRT.

Data Collection

Five data forms were devised. A description of the more significant aspects of the data forms will be given below:

(a) *The presurgical nonradioisotopic data form* contained information on the center and patient identification, on his (her) age and sex, on the past history of nephropathies and occlusive vascular disease, on the blood pressure response to treatment, on plasma creatinine levels and of peripheral plasma renin and renal veins renin (optional). Furthermore, it contained information on renal arteriography (mandatory for each patient included in the study); date of the study, technique (arteriography or subtraction angiography), kidneys' size and location, degree and site of stenosis. In addition, a detailed descriptive angiographic diagnosis and a final extensive diagnostic synthesis and therapeutic decision were collected as a free text.

(b) *The presurgical radioisotopic data form* (and the *postsurgical radioisotopic data form*, for those patients who were submitted to intervention) contained information on the radionuclide tests (performed both without and with captopril 25 mg). ^{99m}Tc-DTPA was suggested as the most adequate tracer. However, it was left free to the individual centers to use hippuran or MAG_3 as a second choice. Attention was given to hydration (8 ml water/kg of body weight in divided doses during the hour preceding dose injection). Antihypertensive medication in the last week preceding the study had to be recorded and was not to be discontinued except for diuretics and ACE inhibitors. Blood pressure measurements were recommended every 15 min after the administration of captopril and at least two measurements had to be recorded respectively before captopril administration and before tracer injection. Captopril (25 mg) had to be given orally 60 min before the injection of the tracer. A warning was given on possible

Table 1. Distribution of patients and major characteristics of the data collected by the participating centers

	AMS	BAR	BOL	BX 1	BX 2	DAN	FRA	GOT	HAM	KUO	LJU	MAC	PAL	PIS	SPJ	STL	ZAG	Total[1]
Number of patients	18	15	116	5	42	6	7	21	7	8	5	16	16	61	14	6	7	370
Diagnostic tests																		
Arteriography	18	5	110	4	4	6	7	20	5	8	4	16	16	44	14	6	7	294
DVSA	–	10	3	1	35	–	–	1	2	–	–	–	–	17	–	–	–	69
RVR	–	–	–	–	5	2	–	8	–	8	3	4	–	16	4	–	6	56
RAS –	13	10	57	–	31	3	–	11	–	3	–	7	8	26	6	4	–	179
RAS +	5	5	59	5	11	3	7	10	7	5	5	9	8	35	8	2	7	191
Tracer																		
DTPA	–	15	110	–	42	5	–	21	7	3	3	16	16	61	14	6	7	326
Hippuran	–	–	–	5	–	1	–	–	–	–	–	–	–	–	–	–	–	6
MAG_3	18	–	6	–	–	–	7	–	–	5	2	–	–	–	–	–	–	38
Intervention	2	1	46	5	–	1	3	4	1	–	1	5	2	18	4	–	4	97
BP outcome	2	1	18	3	–	–	2	–	–	–	–	3	2	17	2	–	–	50

AMS Amsterdam and Rotterdam, The Netherlands
BAR Barcelona, Spain
BOL Bologna, Italy
BX 1 Brussels, Belgium
BX 2 Brussels, Belgium
DAN Danderyd, Sweden
FRA Frankfürt, FRG
GOT Göteborg, Sweden
HAM Hamburg, FRG
KUO Kuopio, Finland
LJU Ljubljana, Yugoslavia
MAC Macerata, Italy
PAL Porto Alegre, Brasil
PIS Pisa, Italy
SPJ St. Priest en Jarez, France
STL St. Leonards, Australia
ZAG Zagreb, Yugoslavia

DVSA = Digital venous subtraction angiography
RVR = Renal vein renin
RAS – = Negative for renal artery stenosis
RAS + = Positive for renal artery stenosis
[1] Data before quality control.

side effects. When present, side effects had to be recorded. Likewise, problems in adherence to the protocol and changes from the standard acquisition protocol of the individual center had to be reported. As concerned the scintigraphic procedure, data were to be acquired and elaborated by a gamma camera-computer system according to the usual protocol for dynamic scintigraphies in use by the individual centers and the choice was given between a series of renal functional parameters to express the final results. The following options were offered: (1) As indices of separate kidney function: renal slopes during the first minutes and/or renal counts during the first minutes and/or initial plateau of the transfer functions (deconvolution analysis). At least one of these three parameters was mandatory. (2) Absolute determination of separate kidney function, overall kidney function and transit times were optional data to be recorded. The choice of the methods was left free and the chosen method had to be indicated. Hard copies of renographic curves and representative images were to be sent with the protocol data. Finally, a strong plea was made that all raw data should be available from long-term storage.

(c) *The postsurgical nonradioisotopic data form* contained information on the date and the technique of vascular repair, on the operative findings, the postoperative status (whether and which control of bypass (or PTA) patency had been made and whether the intervention was not technically successful and why) and on the early follow-up (medication, blood pressure and plasma creatinine values in a control performed 6–12 weeks after the intervention and comments on the clinical success of intervention). Due to their great diagnostic value, every effort was encouraged to collect these data which were to be reported separately and sent later.

(d) *The late follow-up data form* contained information on blood pressure and need for medication during the 6th or the 12th month after intervention which, if available, were also to be sent separately.

Organization and State of the Art

The multicenter study and its protocol were publicized at various scientific meetings of nuclear medicine and hypertension and in several journals of nuclear medicine in the years 1986–1988. A list of potentially interested participants was obtained, to whom a letter was sent. Those centers which were willing to participate in the study were asked to reply with an application form and to send a detailed description of their scintigraphic method. Altogether, 30 centers declared their interest to participate in the study. Up to now (April 1989), data forms of 370 patients were sent by 18 centers. The distribution of patients in the various centers and a few additional major data are reported in table 1. All data forms have been sent to a Central Office (Hypertension Unit, Institute of Clinical Physiology, Pisa, Italy) for review, editing, coding, data entry and analysis. They are checked on receipt for completeness and consistency, queries referred back to local centers for clarification and correction. Overall policy decisions were made by an Executive Committee. Technical assistance was given by L. Mezzasalma for input of raw data on a Macintosh SE Apple personal computer in Excel (Microsoft Co.) files and later transfer on a SPSS file run on a IBM 370 computer, The raw data are currently under review for check of editing errors and quality control (adherence to the protocol, missing or discordant information, consistency of iconographic material, etc.).

References

1 Maxwell MH, Waks AU: Evaluation of patients with renovascular hypertension. Hypertension 1984;6:589–591.
2 NHLBI Workshop on Renovascular Hypertension. Hypertension 1985;7:452–456.
3 Majd M, Potter BM, Guzzetta PC, et al: Effect of captopril on efficacy of renal scintigraphy in detection of renal artery stenosis (abstract). J Nucl Med 1983;24:P23.
4 Wenting GJ, Tan-Tjiong HL, Derck FHM, et al: Split renal function after captopril in unilateral renal artery stenosis. Br J Med 1984;288:886–890.
5 Geyskes GG, Oei HY, Puylaert CBAJ, et al: Renovascular hypertension identified by captopril-induced changes in the renogram. Hypertension 1987;9:451–458.
6 Oei HY, Geyskes GG, Dorhout Mees EJ, et al: The significance of captopril renography in renovascular hypertension. Contrib Nephrol. Basel, Karger, 1987;56:95–103.
7 Fommei E, Ghione S, Palla L, et al: Renal scintigraphic captopril test in the diagnosis of renovascular hypertension. Hypertension 1987;10:212–220.
8 Sfakianakis GN, Bourgoigne JJ, Jaffe D: Single-dose captopril scintigraphy in the diagnosis of renovascular hypertension. J Nucl Med 1987;28:1383–1392.
9 Thorstad BL, Russell CD, Dubovsky EV, et al: Abnormal captopril renogram with a technetium-99m-labeled hippuran homolog. J Nucl Med 1988;29:1730–1737.
10 Dondi M, Franchi R, Levorato M, et al: Evaluation of hypertensive patients by means of captopril-enhanced renal scintigraphy with ^{99m}Tc-DTPA. J Nucl Med, in press.

E. Fommei, MD, CNR–Institute of Clinical Physiology, Via Savi 8,
I–56100 Pisa (Italy)

Blaufox MD, Hollenberg NK, Raynaud C (eds): Radionuclides in Nephro-Urology.
Contrib Nephrol. Basel, Karger, 1990, vol 79, pp 211–218

Captopril Scintirenography: A Protocol to Assess Efficacy and Methodology[1]

A Collaborative Study

Eugene J. Fine

On behalf of The Albert Einstein College of Medicine/Cornell University Medical Center Collaborative Hypertension Group[2], New York, N.Y., USA

Angiotensin-converting enzyme inhibitor (ACEI) scintirenography may reduce the false-positive (FP) and increase the true-positive (TP) rate in the diagnosis of renovascular hypertension (RVH) compared with standard scintirenography, due to a specific renal mechanism of ACEI [1]. Unresolved questions of methodology include choice of radiotracer, patient preparation, timing of ACEI administration, and qualitative versus various quantitative means of study evaluation and processing. Studies aimed at evaluating the TP and FP rate have been reported thus far involving small numbers of patients [2–6].

We are attempting to address these issues of methodology in a 4-year collaborative NHLBI-supported study of two groups of approximately 250–300 patients each. Group A is selected to have a known high prevalence of RVH, to assess the false-negative (FN) rate of ACEI scintirenography. This group is derived from the Cornell University Medical Center Hypertension Clinic (CUMC), a referral base for patients with severe hypertension. Group B is composed of unselected mild hypertensives (DBP 90–100 mmHg) with an expected low (less than 1%) prevalance of RVH to assess the FP rate. This group is composed of patients in an ongoing study of mild hypertension (TAIM) at the Albert Einstein College of Medicine (AECOM).

[1] Supported in part by National Heart, Lung, and Blood Institute, Grant ROI-40566-01.

[2] M.D. Blaufox, MD, PhD (Chairman), E.J. Fine, MD, S. Heller, PhD, S. Mann, MD, T. Pickering, MD, M. Rackson, MD, G. Rottman, MD, S. Sarkar, MD, P. Zanzonico, PhD, C. Zhang, MD.

Methods and Materials

Details of Patient Selection

(a) Assessment of FP rate: As described above, an ongoing evaluation of patients with mild hypertension provides the population from which we anticipate a low prevalence of RVH. Previous studies of similar populations have revealed the prevalence of RVH to be no more than 1% [7]. 250–300 patients will be studied from this population.

(b) Assessment of FN rate: The CUMC will provide patients for the study from two sources. One source consists of patients referred to CUMC with known renal artery stenosis and probable RVH, documented by angiography performed at another institution. These patients will be restudied at CUMC (see study protocol below). On the basis of estimates from prior years, we anticipate approximately 80–100 patients over the next 3 years in this category. In addition, CUMC will provide an additional 100–150 patients (fig. 1). These patients can be expected to have a relatively low prevalence of RVH. The origin of patients arriving in the Nuclear Medicine Department, however, will be unknown to the nuclear medicine staff.

Other Aspects of Patient Selection

Patients in the AECOM group are hypertensive (diastolic BP 90–100 mg Hg), between the ages of 21 and 65 years, and with serum creatinine concentrations less than 2.0 mg/dl. Other exclusions include: pregnancy; a history or other evidence of myocardial infarction during the previous year; stroke; bronchial asthma; diabetes mellitus requiring insulin; allergies to thiazides or beta-blockers; diseases of other major organ systems such as the kidney, the liver; cancer; surgery scheduled or likely during the study period; or life-style or other conditions likely to interfere with adherence to the intervention protocol.

In the CUMC group, subjects will be obtained from two separate sources. In source 1, patients will be selected between the ages of 25 and 70 years with diastolic hypertension above 95 mm Hg off medication. Exclusion criteria include: history within 6 months of myocardial infarction or stroke; diastolic blood pressure greater than 105 mm Hg either off medication or on enalopril or prazosin; serious concurrent illness such as malignancy, anemia, bleeding disorders, etc; poor compliance; mental impairment; or pregnancy. The second source of patients will be referred patients with existing evidence of RVH or renal artery stenosis.

Medication

Patients will be discontinued from all medications consistent with safe medical practice. Continuance of medications will be noted if this is

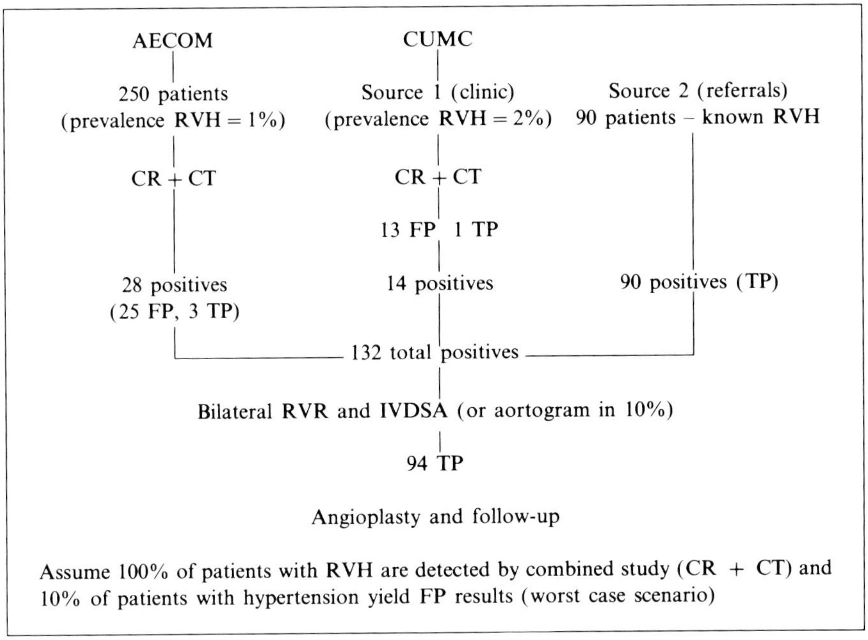

Fig. 1. The flowsheet gives estimates for the AECOM population and the CUMC population. The former has a low prevalance of RVH and as anticipated will provide an estimate of the FP rate of captopril scintirenography. The CUMC population is weighted toward a richer prevalence of RVH and is therefore more likely to provide an estimate of the FN rate. CR = Captopril renography; CT = peripheral captopril renin test; TP = true-positive; FP = false-positive.

required. At minimum, an attempt will be made to remove patients from all diuretics for a period of at least 1 week, from captopril for at least 4 days, and from enalopril for at least 1 week.

Diet and Hydration State

In an attempt to ensure that patients arrive in the Nuclear Medicine Department in a state of 'normal hydration', patients will all be placed upon a 'no salt-added diet'. For some patients this may be an increase in their existing diet and for others a decrease. A no salt-added diet consists of approximately 2–4 g sodium/day. A 12-hour urine collection is obtained and brought to the hospital the day of the scheduled radionuclide scintigraphic exam for assay of sodium, creatinine and volume. A 'spot' collection of urine for specific gravity is also made from a voided morning specimen. Data collection is performed identically at both AECOM and CUMC.

Was patient given 8oz WATER or JUICE prior to radiotracer injections? INDICATE WHICH

POSITIONS	IMAGING, ADMINISTRATIONS AND TRACER INJECTIONS	BLOOD SAMPLES	BLOOD PRESSURES	SUGGESTED TIMER	ACTUAL TIMER	CLOCK TIME	COMMENTS
SUPINE thru 30' Ambulate/Void Y/N ___	First Study I-131-OIH, IV: 150uCi Tc-99m-DTPA, IV: 5mCi			0' 3'	0'		3 ml dose, 10 ml N/S 3 ml dose, 10 ml heparin in N/S
Sit-up 30' thru		5ml green top: ERPF 1st GRF		45'			
		7ml purple top: 1st renin	Base BP1 ___ BP2 ___ Avg ___	60'			
		5 ml green top: 2nd GRF		1 45'			
	Captopril 25 mg in 30 cc H O		Base 0' ___ 15' ___	2:00 2:15			
			30' ___ 45' ___ 1 ___	2:30 2:45 3:00			
3 Hours		5 ml green top: residual bkgd for vitro 7 ml purple top: 2nd renin		3			
	3 min-static bkg image			3:15			8 oz JUICE / WATER to be given; CIRCLE ONE
Supine Thru 30'	2nd Study I-131-OIH, 300uCi Tc-99m-DTPA, 10mCi		BP before sitting up ___	Reset to: 0' 3'	0'		3 ml dose, 10 ml N/S 3 ml dose, 10 ml heparin N/S
Ambulate/Void Y/N ___ Sit up Thur 30'		5 ml green top: ERPF 1st GFR		45'			
		5 ml green top: 2nd GRF		1 45'			
End			Final BP1 ___ BP2 ___ BP3 ___		Discharge:		1) Is patient ready for discharge? Y / N ___ M.D. 2) Total volume N/S administered ___ ml.

Data Collection

The data collection flowsheet is demonstrated in figure 2. In order to assess the virtues of different radiopharmaceuticals, both ^{99m}Tc-DTPA and ^{131}I-orthoiodohippurate (OIH) are used simultaneously. A medium-energy collimator on an Elscint 409AT computer digital gamma camera is employed. The acquisition protocol requires injection of 150 μCi ^{131}I-OIH followed 3 min later by 5 mCi of ^{99m}Tc-DTPA. Acquisition of all data is performed at 3 s intervals for 8 min following injection and at 30 s intervals for an additional 22 min. Digital scinti-images are obtained supine with the camera underneath. The patient is positioned so that an imaginary line between the iliac crests is situated 75 mm above the bottom of the field of view with the aid of a ^{57}Co point source. This ensures position of both kidneys and the heart within the camera field of view. Following completion of acquisition, the patient is seated.

Simultaneous with gamma camera/computer acquisition, in vitro measurements of effective renal plasma flow (ERPF) and glomerular filtration rate (GFR) are accomplished by blood samples obtained 45 min and 1 h 45 min respectively after injection of the radiotracers. The 45-min blood sample is used for calculating ERPF by the method of Tauxe et al. [8, 9]. Use of both blood samples is required for calculation of GFR. While it would be preferable to employ blood samples obtained at approximately 1 and 3 h after injection [10], this would prolong the exam for an unacceptable period of time. Errors introduced by sampling earlier than 3 h will at least be present systematically in samples before captopril as well as after captopril.

After obtaining the second blood sample (1 h 45 min), 25 mg of captopril is crushed and dissolved in 30 ml of water and taken orally by the patient. After a 1-hour monitored interval, repeat computerized scintirenography is performed with 10 mCi ^{99m}Tc-DTPA and 300 μCi ^{131}I-OIH by the identical protocol to the initial study. Repeat blood samples are obtained at 45 min and 1 h 45 min after the second study for post-captopril total renal function measurements.

Simultaneous Stimulated Renin Study

While the patient is seated, a blood sample is obtained prior to the administration of captopril. This serves as a baseline sample for determina-

---

Fig. 2. The flowsheet outlines in compact form the timing and performance of a complete captopril scintirenographic study from administration of ^{99m}Tc-DTPA and ^{131}I-OIH until the completion of the second administration of tracers and the discharge of the patient. The flowsheet serves as a worksheet as well and blood pressure measurements can be recorded as well as the time of entry of all data.

tion of plasma renin activity. One hour after administration of oral captopril, a second blood sample is obtained for determination of stimulated peripheral renin activity.

Patient Monitoring

Patient monitoring is performed after captopril administration at a minimum of each 15 min, for determination of blood pressure response which is noted by the nurse in attendance. A doctor is present for the entire examination.

Centralized Data Collection

All data from CUMC and AECOM is collected on compatible computer equipment. Radionuclide scintirenography data are processed centrally at AECOM after transfer from floppy disks. All patients referred for digital angiography have angiography performed at CUMC where both evaluation and processing of those studies occurs.

Demographic data are entered on a uniform database distributed to both data collection centers and collected at the AECOM, where it is entered into a centralized database by a single individual using widely available software.

Time Allotment for Study Completion (fig. 3)

Nine months were allotted for resolving the captopril renogram method, as described above. From month 9 to month 45, patients are recruited and studied by the prescribed protocol. From month 45 to month 48, data is to be analyzed.

Invasive Diagnosis

All patients with positive criteria for RVH (to be determined) on the basis of scintirenography and stimulated renin tests, or with positive prior angiography, will have digital subtraction angiography (DSA) performed at CUMC with simultaneously obtained individual renal vein renin determinations.

0	9	45	48
Resolve captopril renogram method	Recruit and study patient populations	Analyze data	

Fig. 3. The time of completion of the study is estimated to be 48 months with approximate division of research into sections as schematically outlined.

Processing of Studies

Processing of scintirenographic data is performed at AECOM. Time-activity histograms are derived from manually drawn renal regions of interest (ROIs) and from circumferential background ROIs two pixels away from the renal ROI and two pixels wide for each kidney. From these data, parameters will be derived to characterize renal function and transit. As of this writing, these parameters are being selected from among the following (all derived with and without background subtraction and all pre- and post-captopril): individual percent ERPF and GFR, total GFR, total ERPF, transit time (TT) (DTPA only); time to peak, and percent retention of radioactivity within the kidney at 30 min compared to peak activity. Criteria for a positive study will be determined from the first 20 patients. These criteria will then be used to identify subsequent patients for angiography. Qualitative interpretation will be performed by the principle investigator (M.D.B.). Comparison of qualitative and quantitative interpretation will also be performed.

Discussion

A critical concern in establishing a potential screening exam for RVH is improvement in the specificity, or lowering of the FP rate. Previous studies of standard scintirenography and intravenous urography for screening of a general hypertensive population for RVH indicate specificities in the range of 80–90% [11–15]. The resulting 10–20% FP rate is inadequate when disease prevalence is very low [16].

It is hoped that captopril scintirenography will improve the specificity, lowering the FP rate in the study of patients for RVH. This, however, has not yet been shown in a large series of unselected patients. The objective of the current investigation is (a) to establish uniform criteria of diagnosis and uniform methods, and (b) by study of two large selected populations to establish accurate FP and FN rates in the diagnosis of RVH by captopril scintirenography. This will help clarify the role of captopril scintirenography in the differential diagnosis of RVH.

Relationship to the angiographic standard and to peripheral stimulated renin determinations also will be made. Finally, follow-up of patients will help determine accurate diagnosis of RVH, to supplement the angiographic and clinical diagnosis.

References

1 Hall JE, Guyton AC, Jackson RE, et al: Control of glomerular filtration rate by renin angiotensin system. Am J Physiol 1977;233:F366–F372.

2 Fommei E, Ghione S, Palla L, et al: Renal scintigraphic captopril test in the diagnosis of renovascular hypertension. Hypertension 1987;10:212–220.

3 Sfakianikis GN, Bourgoignie JJ, Jaffe D, et al: Single dose captopril scintigraphy in the diagnosis of renovascular hypertension. J Nucl Med 1987;28:1383–1392.

4 Geyskes GG, Oei HY, Puylaert BAJ, et al: Renovascular hypertension identified by captopril-induced changes in the renogram. Hypertension 1987;9:451–458.

5 Dondi M, Franchi R, Levorato M, et al: Evaluation of hypertensive patients by means of captopril-enhanced renal scintigraphy with technetium-99m DTPA. J Nucl Med 1989;30:615–621.

6 Hovinga TKK, de Jong PE, Piers DA, et al: Diagnostic use of angiotensin converting enzyme inhibitors in radioisotope evaluation of unilateral renal artery stenosis. J Nucl Med 1989;30:605–614.

7 Lewin A, Blaufox MD, Castle H, et al: Apparent prevalence of curable hypertension in the Hypertension Detection and Follow-Up Program. Arch Intern Med 1985;145:424–427.

8 Tauxe WN, Maher FT, Taylor WF: Effective renal plasma flow: Estimation from theoretical volumes of distribution of intravenously injected ^{131}I-orthoiodohippurate. Mayo Clin Proc 1971;46:524–531.

9 Tauxe WN, Dubovsky EV, Kidd T, et al: New formulas for the calculation of effective renal plasma flow. Eur J Nucl Med 1982;7:51–54.

10 Russell CD, Bischoff PG, Kontzen FN, et al: Measurement of glomerular filtration rate: Single injection plasma clearance method without urine collection. J Nucl Med 1985;26:1243–1247.

11 Stewart PH, DeWeese MS, Conway J, et al: Renal hypertension: An appraisal of diagnostic studies and of direct operative treatment. Arch Surg 1962;85:617–636.

12 Wilson L, Dustan HP, Page IH, et al: Diagnosis of renal arterial lesions. Arch Intern Med 1963;112:270–277.

13 Maxwell MH, Goonick HC, Witz R, et al: Use of the rapid sequence intravenous pyelogram in the diagnosis of renovascular hypertension. N Engl J Med 1964;270:213–220.

14 Bookstein JJ, Abrams HL, Buenger RE, et al: Radiologic aspects of renovascular hypertension. 2. The role of urography in unilateral renovascular disease. JAMA 1972;220:1225–1230.

15 Thornbury JR, Stanley JC, Fryback DG: Hypertensive urogram: A nondiscriminatory test for renovascular hypertension. Am J Radiol 1982;138:43–49.

16 Fine EJ, Scharf SC, Blaufox MD: The role of nuclear medicine in evaluating the hypertensive patient; in Freeman LM, Weissman HS (eds): Nucl Med Annu. New York, Raven Press, 1984, pp 23–79.

Eugene J. Fine, MD, Albert Einstein College of Medicine, Department of Nuclear Medicine, 1300 Morris Park Avenue, Bronx, NY 10461 (USA)

Blaufox MD, Hollenberg NK, Raynaud C (eds): Radionuclides in Nephro-Urology.
Contrib Nephrol. Basel, Karger, 1990, vol 79, pp 219–227

Lasix Captopril Renography in the Diagnosis of Renovascular Hypertension

G.N. Sfakianakis [a], *E. Sfakianaki* [b], *J. Bourgoignie* [c,1]

Departments of [a] Radiology (Nuclear Medicine), [b] Epidemiology and Public Health, and [c] Medicine (Nephrology), University of Miami School of Medicine, Miami, Fla., USA

Renovascular hypertension (RVH) is caused by unilateral or bilateral stenosis (fibromuscular or atherosclerotic) of the main renal artery (RAS), branch arterial stenosis, whole kidney or focal renal infarction, aneurysms, and arteriovenous malformations. Clinically, RVH is believed to occur in a subset (1–4%) of the hypertensive population and can be defined as high blood pressure caused by occlusive disease of the renal arterial vasculature, which is potentially curable by surgery (renovascular intervention or nephrectomy), or transluminal renal angioplasty [1]. Renal ischemia due to renal artery or aortic thrombosis in the neonate infant [2] or from iliac artery stenosis in patients with a renal transplant also lead to RVH [3].

Demonstration of causality between the renal arterial lesion and the hypertension is essential to the diagnosis of RVH. Whereas angiography is the gold standard for the diagnosis of RAS, demonstration of an anatomic abnormality does not indicate RVH. Similarly, an angiographic image of RAS does not predict the response of hypertension to renal arterioplasty [1]. Urography (IVP) and conventional, without pharmacologic intervention, radionuclide scintigraphy have an unacceptably high false-negative frequency in diagnosing RVH [1]. Differential renal vein renin determinations are used in the evaluation of RVH, but the test remains invasive and does not provide anatomical information. Measurement of renin activity in peripheral blood before and after captopril is not a specific nor a sensitive test [3].

With curative modes of therapy available, it is important to select and treat those patients with RVH. A noninvasive test sensitive and specific in predicting the outcome of interventional or surgical therapy would be

[1] We would like to thank the Nuclear Medicine Technologists at the University of Miami/Jackson Memorial Medical Center for their work, Dorea Lindo for typing, Pam Little, Chris Fletcher, Douglas Roach and Frynie Sfakianakis for the art work and photography.

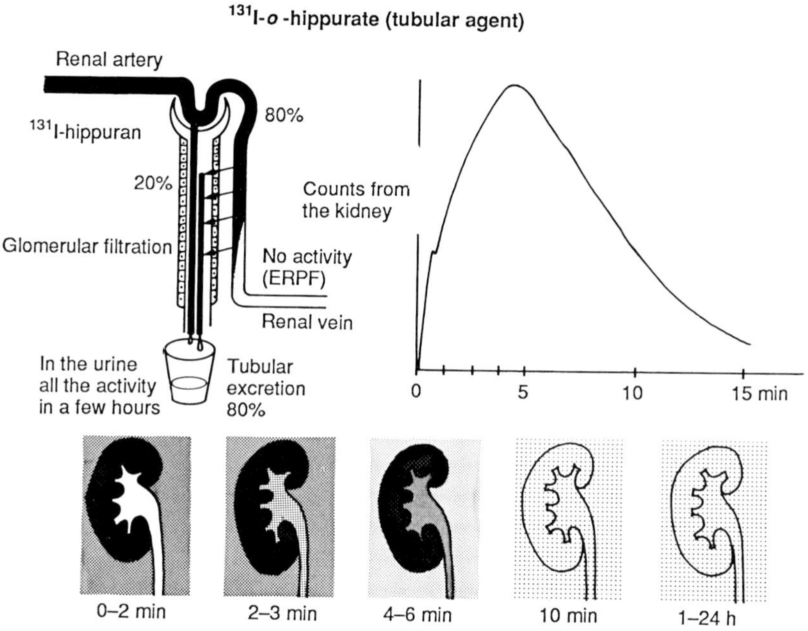

131I-o-hippurate (tubular agent)
Renal artery
131I-hippuran
80%
20%
Glomerular filtration
Counts from the kidney
No activity (ERPF)
Renal vein
In the urine all the activity in a few hours
Tubular excretion 80%
0
5
10
15 min
0–2 min
2–3 min
4–6 min
10 min
1–24 h

1a

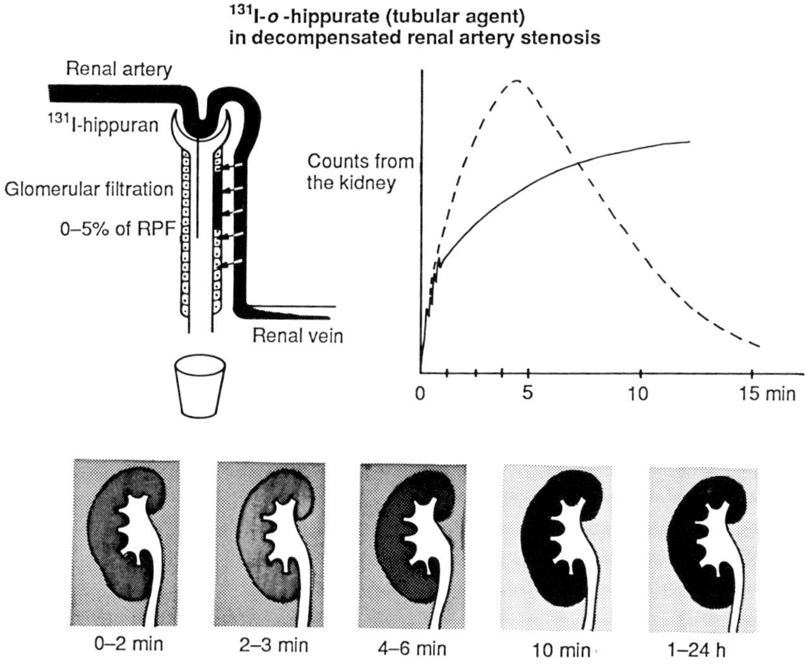

131I-o-hippurate (tubular agent) in decompensated renal artery stenosis
Renal artery
131I-hippuran
Glomerular filtration
0–5% of RPF
Counts from the kidney
Renal vein
0
5
10
15 min
0–2 min
2–3 min
4–6 min
10 min
1–24 h

1b

invaluable for screening and diagnostic purposes [4]. With most other tests yielding less than optimal results, captopril scintigraphy may find a place in this clinical setting [5].

Pathophysiology of Renovascular Hypertension and the Angiotensin-Converting Enzyme Inhibitors

Human unilateral RVH resembles the two-kidney-one-clip model of Goldblatt experimental hypertension; bilateral RVH or RVH from RAS of a solitary (native or transplanted) kidney is comparable to the one-kidney-one-clip model.

A significant RAS, defined as involving more than 60–75% of the lumen of the vessel, decreases afferent arteriolar blood pressure, stimulates pressure receptors, and increases renin secretion by the juxtaglomerular apparatus. A drop in the preglomerular pressure will also decrease glomerular filtration (GF), unless compensation occurs. Indeed, as increased renin is secreted, angiotensin I and (since converting enzyme is present), angiotensin II are locally produced in high quantities; angiotensin II with its preferential action on the efferent arteriole induces postglomerular vasoconstriction, thereby restoring filtration fraction and GF. When angiotensin-converting enzyme inhibitors (ACEI, captopril or enalaprilat) block the production of angiotensin II, post-glomerular vasodilation takes place resulting in a drastic decrease in GF.

The tubular cells in this context retain, at least partially, their functional ability since blood flow to the ischemic kidney is not reduced and may even increase after converting enzyme inhibition. Urine production is decreased or even totally curtailed in the absence of GF. Because of these phenomena, kidneys with RAS following ACEI administration do accumulate tubular agents like ^{131}I or ^{123}I-*o*-hippurate (HIP) or ^{99m}Tc-mercaptoacetyltriglycine (MAG_3) although they do not accumulate glomerular agents like diethylenetriaminopentaacetic acid (DTPA). Since, however, there is not sufficient urine production, the tubular agents (HIP, MAG_3) remain in the cortex of the kidneys for long periods of time (fig. 1a,

---

Fig. 1. a Normal HIP renography. This may be a normal kidney, a kidney with a subcritical ($<70\%$) RAS, or a kidney with compensated significant RAS (80–90%) in a patient with RVH. *b* Abnormal HIP renography (continuous line as compared to normal interrupted line). This can be a captopril-decompensated kidney with RAS 80–95% or a BSL study of a kidney with very severe ($>95\%$) RAS. In the latter case, captopril may further deteriorate the study.

b). Theses effects of ACEI last only a few hours and are totally reversible without residual damage to the ischemic kidney [5].

In contrast, the contralateral nonstenotic kidney in unilateral RVH shows minimal functional changes after blockade of the renin-angiotensin system, and, as long as this kidney is normal, there is no appreciable change in the overall renal function. In bilateral RVH, however, or in a solitary (native or transplanted) kidney with a stenotic artery, and in patients with renal insufficiency and unilateral RVH, ACEI may induce acute renal failure. This side effect lasts while sufficient levels of ACEI circulate. When a single dose of captopril is given for diagnostic purposes, its systemic and renal action last only a few hours, unless severe oliguria is induced, when hypotension lasts longer and recovery of renal function delays for several hours [2].

Severe hypotension may develop as a complication of the ACEI inhibition, even with a single dose of ACEI. This complication occurs in patients with intravascular volume depletion and is responsive to intravenous normal saline infusion. It is advisable therefore, in conducting provocative tests with ACEI, that a vein be available for saline infusion and we advocate the prophylactic use of intravenous saline infusion as will be discussed below. When anuria develops in susceptible patients, administration of vasoconstrictors may rarely become necessary. Angiotensin II is the antidote, a drug very difficult to use and not available commercially [3].

We have introduced the use of furosemide (lasix), which we inject intravenously simultaneously with the tubular agent (HIP) 1 h after an oral dose of captopril [3]. The diuretic is used in an effort to empty the collecting system of the kidney (the pelvis, but mostly the calyces, which extend into the cortex) and increase the accuracy of our approach, which is based on the 20-min cortical residual activity. Furosemide did prevent false-positive studies and, as given in our protocol, acts only by eliminating calyceal and pelvic activity due to its acute diuretic effect [3].

Clinical Experience with Angiotensin-Converting Enzyme Inhibitors (Captopril) Scintigraphy in Renovascular Hypertension

Protocol

Comparative DTPA and HIP studies were performed in our laboratory and results were published before [3]. Since HIP proved to be a superior agent for RVH and after establishing appropriate criteria [6], we introduced the following protocol: Patients should by off ACE Iand all medications should be withheld overnight (for those on ACEI the study is performed without use of captopril). The patient is hydrated (10 mg/kg), and an intravenous infusion of 500 ml normal saline is started slowly at the rate of 4 ml/min. Blood pressure (BP) is recorded,

50 mg captopril (capoten) is given orally, BP is monitored and recorded every 15 min. Scintigraphy is performed 1 h after medication. If BP falls below safe levels, the administration of normal saline is increased (1 liter or more may be required). Most patients receive slowly 500 ml saline. Approximately 5% of patients may need quicker and larger infusions. Out of 300 studies we have observed only 1 newborn baby with bilateral renal ischemia and persistent hypotension after captopril (0.4 mg/kg), who required the use of vasopressor drugs, and 3 patients with orthostatic hypotension at the end of the study, who responded to intravenous saline [5]. Lack of appropriate treatment may cause unwanted complications. Captopril may not be given if the BP is not high enough to allow for a safe reduction for the pharmacologic action of the drug. Anyway, we do not usually give captopril to a patient with a BP below 140 mm Hg.

^{131}I-HIP studies (300 μCi or 11.1 MBq) followed by 40 mg of lasix are conducted in sitting position for 22 min with 2-min images and 30 s per point renograms. Graphs (renograms) for the entire kidney and for the cortex can be analyzed by computing upslope, peak and downslope data; we found it sufficient in the investigation of RVH to compute the percentage of the peak cortical activity remaining at 20 min (residual cortical activity, RCA). When a rising curve ensues, we calculate the percent of peak cortical activity present at 2.5 min postinjection (original cortical activity, or OCA). We suggest the use of lasix (furosemide 40 mg i.v.) at the beginning of the study to induce diuresis and clear the collecting system, thus decreasing the chances of having false-positive studies [3, 5].

Criteria

(a) When the captopril (CAP) RCA is found lower than 30% we report the investigation concluded and not indicative of RVH. When the CAP RCA is greater than 30%, or a rising curve is obtained, we report the study suspicious and recommend a baseline study (BSL) without captopril but with the same protocol, including lasix. For the BSL study, no intravenous infusion of saline is needed. When a BSL shows RCA improvement (10% or more decrease in RCA over the CAP study), the investigation is considered diagnostic of RVH. In all but 1 of 30 proven cases of 70–95% RAS, BSL showed a difference in RCA from CAP renography that exceeded 10% (fig. 2, 3).

(b) When, however, there is too tight a RAS (> 95%), there is only partial or no evident compensation of the renal function by the renin-angiotensin system and BSL and CAP renography are very similar with rising renograms and slight change in the OCA. A rising renogram curve at BSL with little or no deterioration after captopril is therefore considered compatible with RVH.

(c) Finally, when there is angiographic complete obstruction of the renal artery, the kidney is not visualized on ^{131}I renography. Nonvisualization of a kidney, or a part of kidney, is therefore considered compatible with RVH, or branch stenosis, under appropriate clinical conditions.

Findings in Baseline and Angiotensin-Converting Enzyme Inhibitors (Captopril) Scintigraphy

Renographic findings after ACEI depend on the severity of the disease, on the effectiveness of ACEI in decompensating renal function, and on the functional integrity of the kidneys.

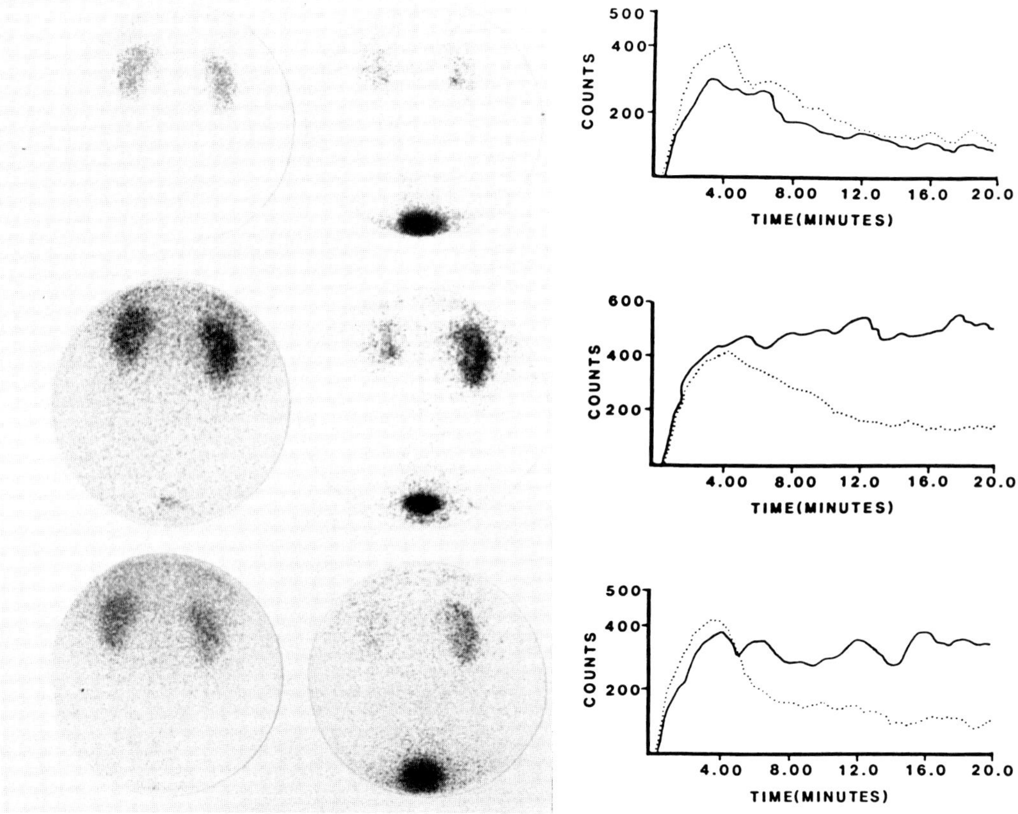

Fig. 2. HIP renography in a patient with right RAS. DTPA studies were borderline positive for RVH. Left: 2 min images; right: 20 min images; upper: BSL study; middle: captopril study; lower: captopril and lasix study.

Subcritical Renal Artery Stenosis (< 60%)

Before clinical hypertension (RVH) develops, approximately 60–75% of the renal arterial lumen must be occluded. Subcritical, asymptomatic RAS in normal kidneys is associated with normal BSL scintigraphy, which is unchanged by ACE inhibition.

Significant (Renin-Angiotensin Compensated) Renal Artery Stenosis (60–90%)

In the presence of a RAS obliterating 60–90% of the arterial lumen, a rather recent onset of hypertension, and an otherwise normal kidney, BSL scintigraphy may be entirely normal; DTPA in typical cases will show

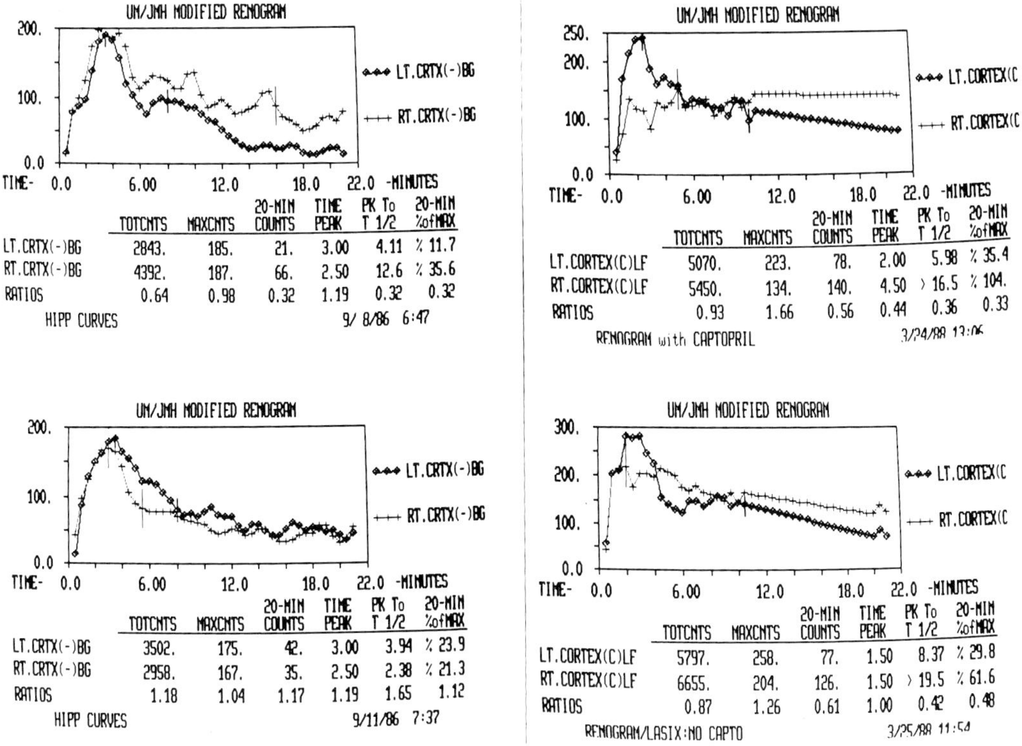

a *b*

Fig. 3. a Cortical renograms with ^{131}I-hippuran (post-captopril, upper; baseline, lower) in a patient with RVH due to unilateral 80% right RAS. DTPA study was negative. *b* Captopril ^{131}I-hippuran renography (upper) in a patient with severe right RAS (> 90%). Notice the abnormal baseline right curve (lower) and the deterioration after captopril (upper). The distal portion of the curves have been manipulated by a least square fitting of a straight line, thus eliminating statistical fluctuations.

a decrease in glomerular function following captopril. With HIP studies, the effect of ACEI is manifested by an early (2–4 min) decrease in activity and by a characteristic, pronounced, cortical retention of the radiopharmaceutical at 20 min, at which time the image of the cortex is prominent and the RCA exceeds 30% of its peak value (fig. 2); in many cases, the CAP renogram shows a late plateau or may be slowly and continuously rising (RCA = 100%) (fig. 2). Usually images at 20 min are more intense than at 4 min.

When renal insufficiency exists, the effects of ACEI are less prominent and difficult to appreciate with DTPA. The same is true in borderline cases (fig. 3a), with a stenosis between 60 and 80%, particularly when there isassociated impairment in renal function. In these cases, HIP has a higher sensitivity than DTPA, because the cortical retention of the activity (RCA) is more easily recognizable and quantitated than a slight decrease in DTPA accumulation [3–5].

Severe Renal Artery Stenosis (> 90%)

As RAS increases from 90 to 95% or more, the BSL renal function may be severely impaired, the kidney shrinks and ACEI effects are less evident. DTPA studies are abnormal, with very low intensity images and suppressed graphs on BSL, and it may be impossible to appreciate any further suppressing effect of the ACEI. HIP studies are abnormal at BSL and there is still deterioration of RCA after captopril (fig. 3b). As the stenosis progresses, BSL is more abnormal and there is little effect of ACEI. Eventually, BSL and ACEI studies are indistinguishable; when renal insufficiency and failure is established, stenotic and nonstenotic kidneys look alike with DTPA. HIP BSL scintigraphy of the severely stenotic kidney is also abnormal, but the abnormality is different from that of the nonstenotic kidney with an identical decrease in renal function: in the RVH-related kidney, cortical HIP accumulates slowly and continuously, unlike in kidneys with other causes of failure, where a low intensity and an early plateauing curve is characteristic. Thus, in extreme cases of RAS, the diagnosis of RVH can be based on BSL findings, even though there may be no appreciable deterioration of I-HIP scintigraphy after ACEI [5]. Of all cases of RVH, only severe stenosis with an abnormal BSL study could be diagnosed by scintigraphy before the introduction of ACEI thereby explaining the low sensitivity of conventional scintigraphy in RVH.

Angiographically Complete Occlusion of the Renal Artery

When RAS progresses to angiographically complete obstruction, the kidney may be kept alive by collateral blood flow; renal ischemia is severe, high levels of renin-angiotensin are produced and RVH ensues. Nevertheless, the kidney is not functioning enough to be visible as a functioning organ on scintigraphy. DTPA may show a trace of flow and faint blood pool activity, which is not modified by ACEI; on HIP scintigraphy the kidney simply does not visualize [3]. Further work is necessary to define the effect of surgical angioplasty in this group of patients. The kidney has developed sclerotic changes and renal parenchymal hypertension is rather predictable. It is doubtful if improvement in renal function and amelioration of hypertension may result from a revascularization procedure [4].

The Newborn Infant and the Child with Renovascular Hypertension

(a) Umbilical artery catheterization may be a life-saving procedure in newborn infants. An occasional complication thereof is aortic thrombosis, which can lead to renal ischemia and RVH because of either impingement of the thrombus on the ostium of the renal artery(ies), or propagation of the thrombus into the renal artery(ies). Kidney ischemia and the hypertension may resolve spontaneously after dissolution or retraction of the aortic thrombus or total destruction of the kidney. Neonates with RVH have been treated with ACEI successfully, but when ischemia was bilateral or associated with a solitary functioning kidney, captopril therapy precipitated renal failure [2]. BSL and single dose captopril scintigraphy with DTPA or GH is important for the diagnosis and prevention of this complication by showing the reversible effect of the single dose [2].

(b) In children and adolescents, we have found single dose captopril scintigraphy with both DTPA and HIP effective in diagnosing RVH; in one patient HIP predicted the results of subsequent angioplasty by showing the effect of ACEI although DTPA scintigraphy did not change after ACEI [5].

Although the method is still under development, it appears that lasix-HIP captopril renography has advantages against DTPA and it is the preferred method, at least until MAG_3 is better studied.

References

1 Madias NE: Renovascular hypertension. AKF Nephrol Lett 1986;4:27–42.

2 Sfakianakis GN, Sfakianaki E, Paredes A, et al: Single dose captopril scintigraphy in the neonate with renovascular hypertension: Prediction of renal failure, a side effect of captopril therapy. Biol Neonate 1988;54:246–253.

3 Sfakianakis GN, Bourgoignie JJ, Jaffe D, et al: Single dose captopril scintigraphy in the diagnosis of renovascular hypertension. J Nucl Med 1987;28:1383–1392.

4 Sfakianakis GN, Bourgoignie JJ, Jaffe D: The effect of captopril on renography in renovascular hypertension (RVH): a predictor of response to angioplasty (abstract). J Nucl Med 1987;28:613.

5 Sfakianakis GN, Sfakianaki E, Bourgoignie J: Renal scintigraphy following angiotensin-converting enzyme inhibition in the diagnosis of renovascular hypertension (captopril scintigraphy); in Freeman LM, Weissman HS (eds): Nuclear Medicine Annual 1988. New York, Raven Press, 1988, p 125.

6 Sfakianakis GN, Fayad F, Ganz W, et al: The advantages of performing captopril scintigraphy before a baseline study in the diagnosis of RVH (abstract). J Nucl Med 1989;30:944.

Prof. G.N. Sfakianakis, MD, Department of Radiology (Nuclear Medicine), D-57, University of Miami School of Medicine, PO Box 016960, Miami, FL 33101 (USA)

Subject Index